The Healing Dance:
A Fusion of Massage & Asian Healing Arts

By *Grace Sunga Asagra MA, RN*

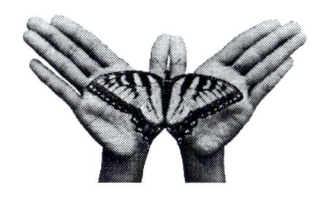

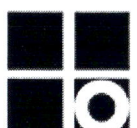

Open Door Publications, LLC

The Healing Dance:
A Fusion of Massage & Asian Healing Arts

Copyright 2014 by Grace Sunga Asagra
ISBN: 978-0996098502

All rights reserved. Printed in the United States No part of this book may be used or reproduced in any manner whatsoever without the written permission of the author except in the case of brief quotations embodied in critical articles and reviews.

The material in this book is not intended as a substitute for advice from physicians, therapists or other professionals. The reader should regularly consult his or her own physician in matters relating to health, exercise, diet or emotional well-being.

Published by
Open Door Publications
2113 Stackhouse Dr.
Yardley, PA 19067
www.OpenDoorPublications.com

Photographs by Ricardo Barros
www.ricardobarros.com/

illustrations by KwaseKhemWer "KK" Asagra Stanley

Cover Painting: Babaylan by Art Zamora

Cover Design by Jessica Chao
www.JessicaChao.com

Dedication   Paghahandog

TO THE VILLAGE
In memory of my father Miguel "Mike" Asagra, sister Ruth "Ruthie" Asagra Stoos, brother Raul "Yoyi", brother Jose "Joe", my grandparents, and my friend, Herbert "Herbie" Tuchman and
To my mother Josefina, aunties, uncles, and cousins
To my sister Edna, sister Patty, brother Timmy, and families
To my son KwaseKhemwer "KK" and family
To African Nganga (Shaman), Akinyele Onisegun Karade, whose indigenous wisdom guided me
To seekers of indigenous-integrative-complementary holistic healing
To friends
To all
To LIFE

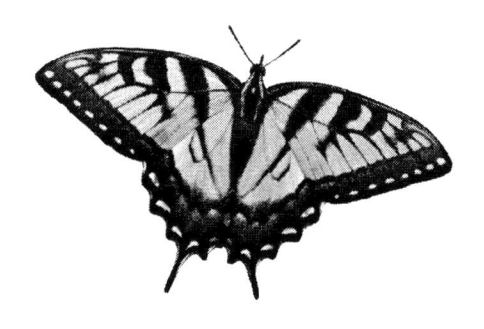

Acknowledgement ᜎᜓᜊᜓᜐ᜔ ᜈᜄ᜔ᜉᜉᜐᜎᜋᜆ᜔ Pagkilala

Lubos po akong nagpapasalamat sa (I am most grateful to):
Diwata (forces in nature) who stay by my side every step of the way,
Ninuno (ancestors) who provide me guidance and protection,
The indigenous healers of the Philippines, Africa, Thailand and other ancient cultures whose universal healing systems live forever,
Mama ko (my mother), Josefina, anak ko (my son), Kwasekhemwer, kapatid kong babae (my sister), Patty, at kapatid kong lalaki (and my brother), Timmy, who shower me with kindness, love and support to follow my dreams,
Willie Stanley and the late Dorothy Stanley, my in-laws, whose love provided me a new family in a foreign land,
Akinyele Onisegun Karade, Nganga (Shaman), for sharing his wisdom of change and transformation,
Hilot students and clients with whom I have experienced teaching and learning opportunities that inspired me to give my best,
The late Herbert Tuchman, whose generosity and friendship were always an incredible support,
Ricardo Barros, versatile photographer, for providing me gorgeous hilot photos,
Jon Bilinski, a kung fu master, who helped me name the photos in this book,
Art Zamora, Filipino modern artist, whose "Babaylan" makes a perfect cover for this manuscript,
Jim, Christopher and Alisson Stoos, my sister Ruth's family, for their love, kindness and generosity,
George Chirco, for holding my hands with patience, perseverance, love and generosity every step of the way,
All my friends and classmates in the Philippines for fantastic memories of growing up, and for supportive friends around the world,
Virgil Apostol Mayor, author of *Way of the Ancient Healer: Sacred Teachings from the Philippine Ancestral Traditions*, for his suggestions, guidance and sincere intent in helping me,
All others whom I failed to mention and yet have supported me in one way or another.
I am deeply in indebted to all of you and it is an honor and privilege to have each and every one of you in my spinning wheel, interwoven in the web of my life.

Disclaimer

Pagtatatuwa

1. This manuscript does not substitute for any study with a Filipino *Hilot or* Thai Massage teacher.
2. This manuscript does not substitute any competent instruction, particularly when it comes to anatomy and physiology.
3. This manuscript does not guarantee safe practice by just reading it.
4. Each receiver is different. Approach can only be customized if the giver is competent and confident as a practitioner.
5. Caution for some techniques must always be observed.
6. Information from this manuscript does not substitute any consultation from physicians.
7. This book serves as a cultural expression of cultural healing.
8. No one owns the truth.

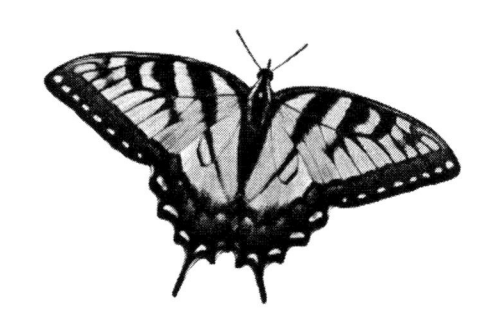

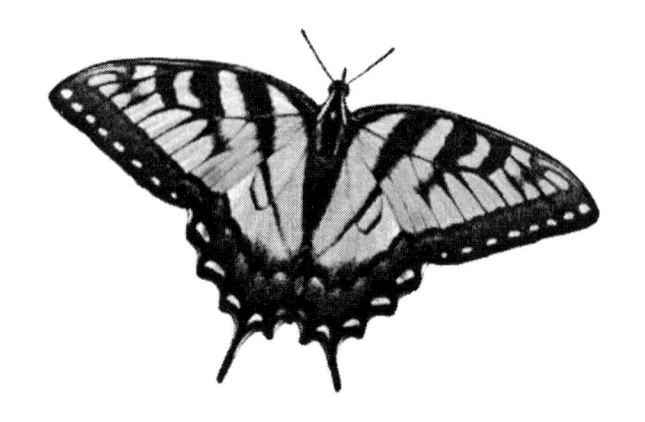

Table of Contents   Talaan ng Nilalaman

Preface *Paunang Salita* 10
Introduction *Panimula* 13
History *Kasaysayan* 17
Salutation *Bati* 20
Benefits of Hilot *Pakinabang ng Hilot* 21
Massage Elements *Kaantasan ng Kaalaman* 22
Cautions *Mag-ingat* 25
Indigenous Advice *Katutubong Payo* 27
Use Your Body *Gamitin ang Iyong Katawan* 28
Basic Dance & Weave *Pangunahing Sayaw at Habi* 30
Introduction to Traditional Thai Massage *Panimula sa Tradisyonal na Thai Masahe* 35
Forces in Nature *Diwata* 92
Recipes *Paraan ng Pagluluto* 98
Poems *Tula* 105
What's Next? *Ano ang Susunod?* 110
References *Mga sanggunian* 112

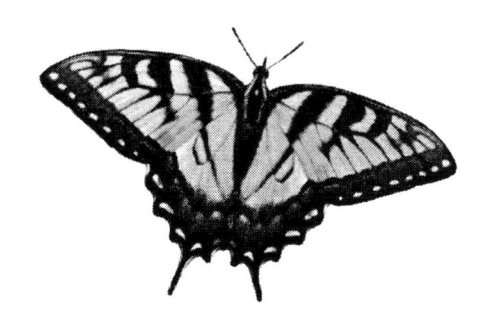

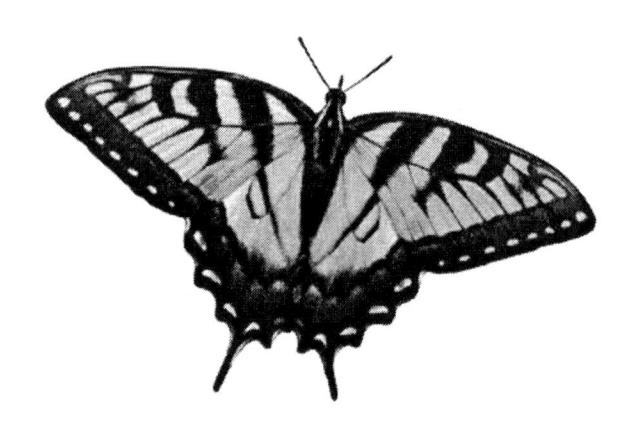

Preface
Paunang Salita

Traditional indigenous healing is abundant in the Philippines. I grew up in the Bicol Region, which is located in Southern Luzon where I was blessed to have mingled with parabulong (healers) of all kinds—hilot (massage therapists), arbularyo (herbalists), and espiritista (shamans), just to name a few.

What's fascinating about these healers is that each is gifted with the knowledge, skills and wisdom to use a combination of techniques to facilitate healing, expanding the responsibility of the hilot who uses his or her skills so others can be helped in their acute or chronic health issues. To address the symptoms, a hilot addresses emotional, mental, nutritional, behavioral and spiritual factors that influence health and wellness.

The word hilot translates to mean the person doing healing, the techniques used in healing, as well as the actual healing itself. It's one of those Filipino words that is not easy to define with just one word, as there are several possible meanings, particularly in relationship to Filipino healing arts. After all, what's a word without the experience?

I treasure the experiences I had growing up with hilot, learning from my mother, Josefina, and my auntie, Peling. My late grandmother, Lola Julia, was an arbularyo who took care of some of my cuts and scrapes with various herbs. I remember her chewing betel nut leaves and lime and packing it on my finger to heal a cut draining with pus. Every now and then a well-known hilot would come to our house when someone was really sick, or we would go to an arbularyo in remote areas.

Although it is still practiced throughout the Philippines, many people who are influenced with Western ways now consider herbal healing superstitious and backward. This was not the case in our household, where indigenous ways were our first aid resource as well as an alternative resource when other modern ways of healing did not seem to work. We did not have health insurance to use for medical doctors, something I now think of as an advantage, since we learned to use local resources of herbs, foods and ways that are now accepted as complementary and integrative. Bitter melon and moringa, commonly eaten and growing wild in the Philippines, are in the list of ingredients of nutraceutical products today.

It was in the 1980s that I truly began to see the importance of our indigenous healing arts and how they are related to all healing arts in Asia. As I learned from local hilot/arbularyo and ordinary folks, I felt so much appreciation

The Healing Dance

for my culture and all the mystical powers that come with it. I knew then that it touched a very deep part of my soul.

Filipino healing art dates back to the pre-colonization period, and is a combination of varied cultural influences introduced through trading and migration amongst, to name just a few, Asian, Polynesian and Indo-Melayu kingdoms and nations. I took great pride as I learned of this part of my heritage. This conglomeration of healing practices that evolved from the country's history is a fusion of Asian healing arts.

When I came to the United States in 1985, I was fascinated to see all the sophisticated herbal stores where herbs are packaged neatly and kept in decorative jars. At that time, all I did in the Philippines was pick the herbs and dry them under the sun. It was also surprising for me to learn that there were massage schools in the United States, and that it took a paper of completion, a certificate of training or a license to give a massage. On the other hand, I have always looked at our hilot in the Philippines as gifted and spiritual practitioners from lineages whose process in learning to practice healing was culturally different. I asked myself the question, "What role do I have in healing?"

I hesitated to share publicly my knowledge of indigenous healing until I got sick in the summer of 1996. My body was covered with boils. I could not even expose my arms and enjoy the sunshine. I was very restless, and deep in my heart I knew I would like to incorporate hilot and other indigenous healing arts in my practice in United States. "How can I heal myself?" I asked. This question reminded me of what my teachers always said: "Know thyself to heal thyself."

This is where the "fun" begins in my own journey with a shaman whom I met in the United States. At the time, I felt as if the full moon was shining right at me in the darkest moment when I came to understand, to take courage, to be humble and honor mystery. My shaman teacher has a gift of seeing things and making sense of them. With his help, I realized that I have the gift of healing from my culture. After trying other things to make myself better, I turned to my cultural traditions. Out of this experience, I came to realize that my boils were no different from my desires trying to ripen and come out of my system, my hesitation, my doubts and my fears. I just said the words, "Okay, I am going to do it and I will be helped by the diwata (spirits/angels/forces in nature) and mga ninuno (ancestors)." Then I had so much joy using herbs and medicinal foods to help me. It was a home away from home. My whole body started to heal in less than a week.

Filipino hilot was not well-known in the United States when I made this decision. Thai massage had just begun to be popular. Through Thai massage I felt closer to my Asian roots. I found a gateway to Asian fusion healing that opened for me to seek out connections to other Asian healing arts such as Ayurvedic and Chinese massage.

In this book, I am honoring the Thai massage techniques that I have blended with my background in hilot because they are so similar to the techniques that I grew up with. Unlike Thai massage, which has been documented for preservation, Filipino hilot is a dominantly oral tradition, practiced mainly by traditional practitioners. Doing hilot since the 1980s, I am inspired to continue to share my cultural expression of healing in ways that are dear to me as I pay homage to my ancestral lineage. Of course, with my son as the co-creator in this book, it also becomes a personal legacy that I leave for my family, my people and others.

The vision of this book came in the middle of the night as I was sleeping. Dreams are regarded as communications with the diwata. I envisioned a manual rich in illustrations and practical directions so that even a child would want to read and learn from it. At the same time, each page would reflect the warmth, nurturing and power of hilot. It is also my intention that the book will be a guide easily understood by seekers and learners.

Let there be silence and surrender to pulsations of natural rhythm—simple yet complex, unique but common—that resonate and can connect us to kaluwalhatian (peace), kalusugan (health), ugnayan (relationships) ligaya (joy) and kaligtasan (safety).

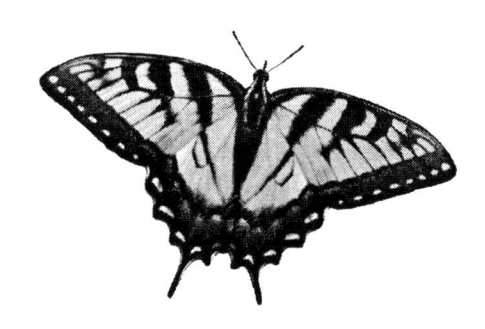

Introduction   Panimula

Allow me to lead you on an enjoyable journey all the way to ancient Asia. It is a path of healing-in-progress where your heart is in a harmonic convergence of your truth—your own experience, not that of anyone but you. It is a dance that touches you from the very depth of your being to the crown of your spirit. The dance may be in private. The dance takes place on the external visible level, but is richly connected on the internal invisible level. This is where healing begins.

Consider this book as a cultural expression where bridges are formed for healing. It invites you to cross over from illness to wellness by looking at the roots of the illness, instead of avoiding them. It motivates you to establish trust with your dance partner for health promotion, restoration and sustenance in an on-going healing work that finds meaning in the discomforts, ailments, emotions, pains and sorrows embodied in our bodies and behaviors. It is in dancing that we can connect with our bodies, notice our limitations and recognize them not as restrictions, but bridges to healing.

For the inspiration that I generated from Thai healing arts, I felt compelled to feature a dance with you through photographic and instructional techniques as an introduction to Thai massage, which I have closely interwoven with my Filipino hilot practice. While I did not address specific ways to manage common symptoms and incorporate medicinal herbs used in hilot, it is my vision that you will explore those possibilities as you progress. There is no one way, one solution, even for the same ailment. Take the opportunity to study with a teacher.

In honor of my Filipino ancestors, I offer thanks in Tagalog, one of the Filipino languages as inscribed in Baybayin, our pre-Hispanic Filipino script. In respect to Thai healing traditions, I also included a Thai prayer I learned in the course of my studies. Thoughts of gratitude are part of the dance invitation for the energetic presence of those who have come before us in this time of knowing. Practice of gratitude is humbling and respectful, and sets a good tone for a harmonious dance.

You can't have a good dance without music. Music in the form of proverbs, poems and words of caution is equally important to the joint-muscular manipulative techniques. In the massage technique section, while the giver and the receiver enjoy the dance, both travel to a space and time that speaks of the way a group of people value time and health as very precious in their lives. In the East, it is not unusual to have a massage for three to four hours. In the West, almost everything is about how fast we can accomplish our long to-do lists and our hard-driven goals. Long hilot sessions can help you to be in the moment, in deep relaxation and meditation. Breathing is soft and peaceful. Journalist and essayist Henry Louis Mencken states, "Time is the greatest equalizer."

The benefits of hilot that I listed at the beginning are not limited to that list. You can add more as a living witness to healing. The dance experience can mean different things to different people. Although the dance is experienced in the moment, the power of the dance is in its partnership work, and it is always a work in progress.

This practice requires the practitioner to be in good health, "physician, heal thyself," so to speak. This compelled me to write a section on the characteristics of a successful practitioner as well as cautions to take in hilot sessions. Don't add more to any injury. If you are in the healing business, manifest health that will provide a good impact on those around us. This also brought me to include a section on the use of the whole body in this practice, as exemplified in Filipino martial art that is integral in many aspects in the culture.

Hilot and Filipino martial art known as kali, arnis, or eskrima in most parts of the Philippines and silat in Muslim population in the Southern Philippines, are closely related. In hilot as in kali and other Asian martial arts, before you become an instructor, you have to know how to heal yourself. Kali, in its dance form, includes knowing when to use various parts of the body. There are many technical movements, termed locks and holds in martial arts, which are used in hilot. Both hilot and kali require whole body attention and focus for the dance to work without hurting anyone. You can use the same movement or part of the body to hurt or heal. Interestingly, most good martial artists are also good dancers.

Ancient cultures recognized and understood the seen and unseen world. They had no doubts that energies or spirits exist and influence everything in life. To Filipinos, awareness in diwata (forces in nature) and ancestral energies was fused in everything. Their guidance was understood and influenced people's health, livelihood, harvests, life, sickness, death and reincarnation.

The diwata naturally occur in nature. Their purpose is to live in harmony with anything and everything. Disharmony in nature creates disharmony in the body. This can lead to unpleasant circumstances. The on-going process of seeking harmony continues in daily life. Everything is considered medicine. The healers bridge the gap between nature and humans.

Although the majority of Filipinos are now Christian, the earlier peoples also practiced indigenous rituals. Some were Hindu, Buddhist and later Muslim (the latter still prevalent among some southern ethno-linguistic groups). Many, however, still practice and respect diwata as an intimate part of our indigenous culture. The last time I was home, my uncle, who is a Christian, was offering thanks and asking permission from the diwata in the bananas when we picked some leaves.

There is a correlation between the diwata and the chakra philosophy in yogic traditions, and with African deities. The diwata are as much as a part of the human body as they are a part of nature, as taught in yoga, kali, and traditional dances. I have included a brief explanation of chakras (diwata) to reinforce healing by looking inside ourselves as opposed to looking outside of ourselves for cause and solutions. Afrikan Nganga (Shaman) Akinyele Onisegun Karade once said, "Things that we take in or do in defense against the enemy thinking that our enemy causes our misery and make us sick, we have to look into the inner me."

As to techniques, each can be revised according to the need of the receiver. The whole process can be shorter or longer. Although this is dominantly hands-on practice, a situation may call for less of hands-on. Done in slow motion as traditionally practiced, this is not all about constant movements. The pause can bring out a mindful healing that may just be what's needed. The healer is the conduit for this process to take place even after the session.

Hilot is applicable for the wellness of all ages. It was deemed necessary to see a hilot or invite a hilot to come to the house to bring comfort to the sick through his or her presence and healing hands. There is a general impression that a hilot is old. In our culture, old age means seasoned skills and wisdom.

In indigenous cultures, being of largely an oral tradition, we grew up learning about life as we live it and from conversations that are coated with many salawikain o kasabihan (proverbs or sayings). This is part of the dance music. We hear them from our parents, grandparents, uncles, aunties and the elders. It is not necessary to share a common bloodline because everyone in the community is "related." When we are in the presence of an elder, our responsibility is to listen to stories, proverbs, parables, jokes and songs. Since education takes place through listening, I included a few kasabihan (sayings), tula (poems), and kwento (short stories) that are applicable to this book. They are music to my ears. The poems I included are poems of healing and friendship. This also reminds me of the use of chants, still a form of music in indigenous healing in Asia, Africa and Polynesian culture.

What would cultural dance expression be without food shared or offered? I have included paraan ng pagluluto (recipes) of food for healing. Asia is a wealth of natural resources for economic growth, community development, sustenance and health. If there is no disparity in economic wealth and power, no Asian, children in particular, will go to sleep hungry, nor die in hunger.

Indigenous healing traditions remind us that experience precedes knowledge. What makes the hilot powerful is that it can incorporate anything from around the world. Hilot becomes inclusive of all healing arts: place it in one pot, let it brew and make it work.

This dance is as meditative as it can possibly be while also being a reflection of an ancestral "tapestry." Each movement contributes to an actual process of textile, life making that spins (rotations, flexions, extensions), dyes (use of herbs), weaves (rocking, pressing, rolling, pulling, patterns), embroiders (use of fingers, thumb, knees, circles) and tailors (sensitivity, consciousness, compassion) the fabric of healing in the web of life. The giver and the receiver are unique strands chosen for the particular occasion to be worn in harmony with the universe.

Physical space and privacy is never an issue in the Philippines, Thailand or other countries in Asia. People don't mind being physically close to each other. We even have a joke that in a straw mat measuring six feet by twelve feet, fifty people can sleep, as long as they are in a vertical position. Each moment is considered sacred but not isolated to our day-to-day life. When Asian friends and relatives come to visit one another in United States, where they sleep is not a concern. Every inch of floor has the potential to be a bed. We can both laugh and cry at the same event. We don't have to be quiet to do the massage. As the process progresses, we continue to connect with one another. Provided both the giver and the receiver are comfortable, it is not required to have a special mat. The receiver is lovingly cared for as the giver cuddles the inner child of the receiver.

I observed that a Thai cultural practitioner does not spend too much time in labeling a style of Thai massage, whether it is northern or southern style or whether it be first, second, third or fourth level. Thai massage just is. Filipino hilot is the same. Besides, hilot in its fullness is hard to describe in words. A technique of the hilot is open for modifications as the situation calls for it, and flows with the receiver's body. In the end, the dancing and weaving is completed, leading to a connection between one another and the entire web of creation.

As we patiently travel toward a wonderful experience, let us explore and experience that which is meaningful within the differences and similarities in cultures around the world. Healing, as my teachers say, is not so much what we learn but what we have unlearned. Above all, let us pay due homage and respect to the people in Asia for sharing their healing treasures.

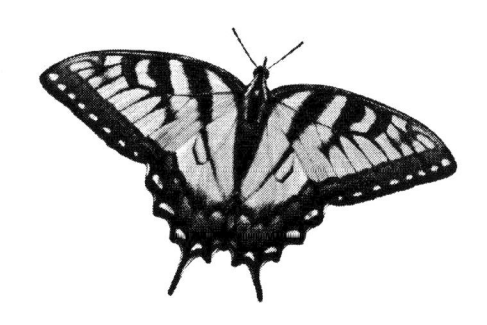

History   Kasaysayan

I bring forth to you the kasaysayan coming from the Filipino oral tradition of story-telling transcribed to share with the modern world of dominantly written tradition. Here I gracefully begin:

The origins of Filipino hilot, Thai massage and other Asian indigenous healing arts are not easy to trace because these civilizations pass on their history primarily through oral traditions. However, the Philippines has Baybayin, an ancient pre-colonial writing system, written on impermanent "pads" such as leaves, tree branches and trunks. Most details of the ancient history in Thailand and other Asian countries is believed to be in Grantha, a palm leaf writing of the Pallava era between the Second and Ninth Centuries. The Philippines and many nations in Asia were known as one large kingdom, not as the different nations we currently know. There is one popular belief that warlike nations destroyed many palm leaf writings. Another belief is that the information written on perishable materials just deteriorated due to high heat and humidity. Whatever is left of Thailand's shared written history was carved in stones.

In addition, as part of the systematic strategies of control, power and greed, colonizers imposed their own ways of writing and speaking, perpetuating abuse by the ruling class and foreign domestic rulers during the colonial system. Ethnic cultures were systematically destroyed. Propagation and preservation of healing arts were challenged as people were displaced constantly by political, economic, and socio-cultural conditions. Although I have found a scarcity of writing on hilot, I have observed hilot as a thriving practice to this day in the Philippines and other nations where Filipinos are living. The hilot ancestral lineage is honored by those who live their purpose as hilot. When they do this, they bring with them the entire healing lineage of those who have come before them.

In the deep rural areas it is common to have a member in the family who knows some basic techniques in healing such as basic massage techniques or common herbs for common ailments. But hilot is a specialized field that comes directly by birth, direct experience and training. If you're not born with it, it's not happening. Certain aspects can be taught to others. Others are difficult to explain in words.

Ancient cultures around the world were immersed in nature beyond what the eyes can see. The tangible means of healing came not just from earth's resources, but also from the awareness that there is an on-going infinite connectivity of all creations in the universe. Practicing elders of the ancient healing arts acknowledged with humility their role in healing. They were respected and honored as masters in ancestral healing arts.

Filipino healing arts has its geographical roots in the Philippines in relation to ancient Asia and the ancient global trading system. Think of it as an old tree with many big roots growing in all directions, deeper, wider and only sometimes seen on the surface. Yet, what you see is nothing when compared to what you do not see. The root system of the tree is a mystery in the vastness, expansion, and weaving that goes on underneath the tree. The power of an old tree is not how tall or wide it is, but the infinite symbiosis and synergy of the dance in the roots. A tree is that which connect us to earth and to the universe.

All indigenous healings, like trees, are interconnected in their roots so it is not surprising to notice similarities such as use of plants to heal, honoring ancestors, calling upon diwata (forces in nature), and adequate rest to recover from any ailment. It is like the neuron networks in our system: if there is disconnect, or if the synapses are not talking to each other, disharmony (illnesses, depression, anger, etc.) is bound to happen, and harmony is challenged. Indigenous healing such as hilot acknowledges the unity in healing instead of compartmentalizing things; it is viewed as a whole. It does not cause alienation. It is integration and promotes communication.

Filipinos from all walks of life acknowledge the role of hilot as an intervention for a variety of health conditions from chronic (i.e. joint pain, fatigue, difficulty in pregnancy) to acute (i.e. sprain, broken bones). Hilot is affordable, familiar, practical, effective and accessible. Hilot is a practice that goes beyond bone, or musculo-skeletal manipulation. Herbs, foods, relationships and behaviours are addressed. It is open for possibilities of sustainable health that is authentic and bio-individual. Conversations with Filipinos and other immigrants in the United States share successful health stories using cultural interventions such as familiar herbs for headache or the bentusa technique.

Bentusa (cupping) is an indigenous healing art popular in the Philippines, China and other Asian countries. Herbs such as ginger are sliced into small round pieces, placed on the person's affected area and the small glass cups are heated and placed over the ginger. This practice was recommended to alleviate pain and inflammation, remove toxins and promote relaxation.

Ancient kingdoms shared common experiences of authentic originality, growth, exploitation, exploration, indigenous medicines, foods, herbs, plants, dances, music, chants, martial arts, animals, tools and other resources for survival and progress. Filipinos in, their own autonomy prior to modern history, welcomed all traders, resisted invaders and ferociously fought colonizers. In spite of the abuse, Filipinos remained trusting and compassionate to those who came from other cultures. Women played major roles in maintaining the culture. According to traditions, the diwata in charge of maintaining the culture is female.

There are stories that as the monks and nuns traveled around Asia, particularly Thailand, they brought the healing art of massage to help people go into deeper meditation. That's why in the early years, Thai massage was administered only in temples. This style of massage flourished in Thailand and its basic set of movements and motions have endured. It was not until the late 19th century that it began to spread in the community outside the temple to become part of the folk medicine of the Thai people.

So, in ancient cultures, when it comes to concerns of the body, the intervention goes beyond manipulation, pressure points and other massage techniques. It is easier to name it as massage, but the deeper connection of the modality is intended to address the roots of the problems. This is where the dance begins, with specialists in the field as the healing dance teachers.

The Western influence has greatly diminished the use of traditional healing. But with the current increase in chronic health conditions, stressful demands of work and raising families, longing for self-care, and wanting to belong, there has been an increasing interest in studying and rendering massage at homes, and in the community at large. For some, temples remain the main centers for education and healing while others seek cultural practitioners who live their purpose as hilot.

Hilot honors touch as a healing therapy. Touch is crucial in all living beings particularly the young. For humans, touch started in the womb. It's been said orphans left in cribs die not of infections in a very sterile field, but from touch deprivation. Studies in animals deprived of touch showed poor growth and poor survival. Skin is directly connected to the nervous system. Hilot provides an opportunity for sensitivity training similar to martial arts training. Locks and hold motions provide information of relaxation and letting go. It is not just to know the techniques, but to be aware of surroundings. Adults who are touched deprived misinterpret touch when hilot is in progress. It is important to have respectful intentions of both giver and receiver. This honors those who have paved the way for a sacred cultural healing expression.

Wherever we are, we can always go back to our roots, calling a whole army of ancestors and healing traditions. It is the wellspring where we can quench our thirst for authentic knowledge, inspiration, support and love. As the wise say, "The wheels are already invented." We do not have to rediscover it, but we can enhance it. Our roots are available for us to explore authentically.

There are hilot cultural health practitioners who have dedicated their lives to cultural preservation. As ancestral tradition bearers, they are consciously aware of the interconnectivity of anything and everything in the matrix of the web of healing. Ancient healing arts will be shaped by those who practice and experience them. It will not be defined by mere techniques. Instead, it will be defined as an integration of all-inclusive healing arts responsive to the needs of the times. Indigenous healing such as hilot will continue to find its role in health and wellness as healing fusion continues.

Salutation

Bati

PRAYER I CREATED FOR MY HILOT PRACTICE
Lubos po akong nagpapasalamat
Sa mga biyaya na ibinigay niyo sa amin
Sa oras pong ito, basbasan niyo ang aming kalusugan

I am forever grateful
For the blessings you have given to us
In this moment, please bless our health

PRAYER I LEARNED FOR THAI MASSAGE
(Used with permission: Institute of Thai Massage, USA)
Om namo Shivago silasa ahang
Karuniko sapasatang osatha tipa mantang
Papaso suriya-jantang. Gomalapato paka-sesi
Wantami bantito sumethaso Arokha sumana-homi

(Repeat the above three times)

Piyo-tewa manussanang piyo-proma namuttamo
Piyo-nakha supananang pininsiang nama-mihang
Namo Putaya navon-navien nasatit-nasatien
Ehi-mama navien-nawe napaitang-vien
Navien mahaku ehi-mama piyong mama namo-puttaya.

Na-a Na-wa rokha payati vina-santi.

(Repeat final line three times)

We invite the spirit of the Founder, the Father, Doctor Shivago, who comes to us through his saintly life. Please bring to us the knowledge of all the nature that this prayer will show us, the true medicine of the Universe. In the name of this mantra, we respect your help and pray that through our bodies you will bring wholeness and health to the body of the one we touch.
The Goddess of Healing dwells in the heavens high, while mankind lives in this world below. In the name of the Founder, may the heavens be reflected in the earth below so that this healing medicine may encircle the world.
We pray for the one whom we touch, that illness may be released and that happiness will follow.

Benefits of Hilot Pakinabang ng Hilot

Deep Relaxation
Very comforting and nurturing
Relieves pain
Reduces stress
Improves circulation
Enhances flexibility
Stabilizes mobility
Releases toxins
Improves internal organ functions
Builds up immune system
Realigns body
Re-energizes all the chakras
Balances all the elements
Reconnects with the deities
Awakens and elevates consciousness
Makes us feel pampered
Harmonizes the body's rhythms to the Universe
And more

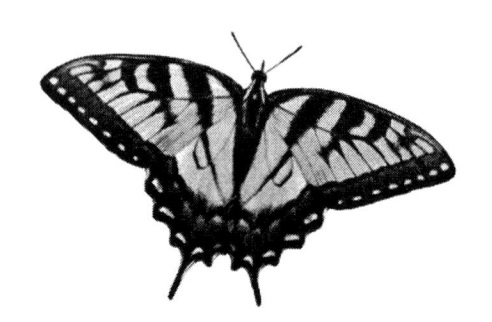

Elements / Elemento

An effective nurturer goes beyond the attainment of knowledge of techniques and motions. A good nurturer is the embodiment of health, discipline and compassion. How good you are depends upon how much of yourself you give during a never-ending training process.

Many elements beyond technique can be taken into consideration. I have listed seven of them below, along with some Filipino idiomatic expressions and proverbs that help me to remember that these elements are key.

KALAKASAN (VIGOR for Stamina and Endurance)
Magtipon ng lakas. (Gather your strength)

Vigor is the driving force to have the stamina and endurance. This work is very physical and could give the nurturer a feeling of fatigue and exhaustion. A healthy lifestyle contributes to not just the physical strength needed but to the unwavering inner strength grounded in truth and principles of healing.

INSPIRASYON (INSPIRATION for Confidence)
Ang nakikinig sa sabi-sabi ay walang tiwala sa sarili. (When you listen to hearsay, you have no confidence in yourself.)

The inspiration coming from your instructor, your clients and your techniques will help you in what you are doing and gain confidence. But above all, the inspiration (in-the-spirit) from within, will give you confidence, and with it humility.

KATATAGAN (STABILITY for Coordination)
Tinimbang ka, ngunit kulang (When weighed, found wanting)

Stability through harmony of mind, body, emotions and spirit will lead you to balance the weave of every motion you decide to do, whether it is a pattern or an addendum to the routine. It is important to spend time and energy tending to all areas and aspects of compassion that matters for the individual.

PAGLINGAP (NURTURING for Refinement and Style)

Nasa tao ang gawa, nasa Diyos ang awa. (In a person who works, God has mercy.)

Nurturing can bring out the best in oneself. Without the Divine's omnipresence, omnipotence and omniscience in our being, techniques will remain techniques rather than instruments of healing. Your own style and system unfolds with God's grace and through diligence and practice.

SIMBUYO NG DAMDAMIN (PASSION for the Work)
Buhos na kalooban (Unconditional commitment)

Passion for growth, for success, for excellence through one's determination and love of the work can only come from belief in oneself, leaving no room for any doubt or fear. Doubt and fear can only lead to lack of commitment and focus. When you love something, it brings about transformation and unity with yourself, your clients and the spirits of the ancient healing arts. Yearning leads to the desire for knowledge to understand the interrelationships of techniques, patterns, things and events in the dance as it's woven in the web of life.

PAGIGING ISA (ONENESS for Sensitivity and Awareness)
Ang taong hindi marunong lumingon sa pinaggalingan ay hindi makakarating sa kanyang paroroonan. (If you don't look at where you came from, you will never be able to reach your destination.)

Everything is medicine wrapped in gratitude. Our past, our present and our future come with medicine needed at the right moment as we look into our habitual patterns that may cause joy and sufferings. They are the roots that keep us growing. We cannot deny events that have happened, or emotions felt in our life's journey. Understanding and appreciating all moments help us to be one with ourselves, our clients and all our surroundings. Being one increases our keenness and sensitivity to forces in nature. It gives us clarity and direction. It sharpens our listening abilities beyond what we only want to hear. It helps us notice things to which we normally would not pay attention. Our senses become a source to protect ourselves from harm's way. To be one is to listen with our hearts as compassion unfolds healing. Be grateful, relax your whole body, stay calm and be alert. Be ready to attune yourself to the unfolding dynamic.

KABANATAN (RESILIENCE for Patience, Trust and Faith)
Kapag may tiyaga, may nilaga. (When there is patience, something is brewing.)

Resiliency is empowered through patience, trust and faith. We are called to give way to the master plan of diwata. Be harmonious with the forces in nature. This will allow us to enjoy a delicious dish of health and well-being. Be like the water. Transform as you flow. Helping others calls us to re-shape ourselves in many ways necessary to create harmony and yet remain true to our being.

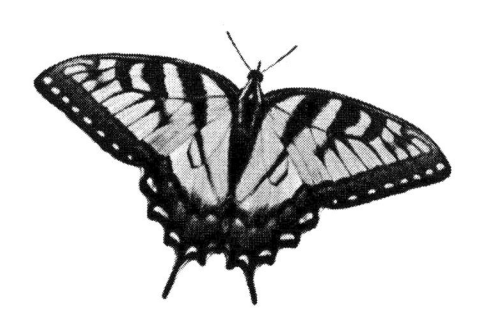

Cautions   Mag-ingat

1. Do not do hilot on a FULL STOMACH or a FULL BLADDER. Abdominal massage, lower body twists and pressure points might cause discomfort.

2. During PREGNANCY, do not do the hilot during the 11th, 12th and 13th weeks. In case of complications and previous history of miscarriage, ask receiver to seek medical advice. Do not perform any move that will constrict the abdomen. Do not put heavy pressure on the sen lines (energy lines). Please remember, two lives are involved. You just want to support the pregnancy process, not alter it. Seek advice unless you have the training and experience to deal with this situation.

3. Do not do hilot immediately following SURGERY. Seek advice unless you have training and experience in the situation.

4. In the event of JOINT PROBLEMS, advise the receiver to seek medical advice. Use slower, softer techniques and extra support during rotation, pressing, stretching and pulling. Seek advice unless you have training and experience in dealing with this situation.

5. If the receiver is FATIGUED or BREATHLESS, ask him to seek medical advice. Movements must be slower and softer. Position the receiver so that there are no restrictions on the chest. If needed, elevate the head. Seek advice unless you have training and experience in dealing with the situation.

6. During MENSTRUATION, avoid heavy pressures on the sen lines. Moves that raise the legs over the head must be slower and less frequent. Once legs are over the head, do not hold the position.

7. For those who have HEART CONDITIONS, ask receiver to seek medical advice. Moves that raise the legs over the head must be slower and less in frequent. Once legs are over the head, do not hold the position. Do not hold the brachial and femoral pulses for more than five seconds. Seek advice unless you have training and experience in dealing with the situation.

8. For SKIN PROBLEMS, ask receiver to seek medical advice. The giver must clean her hands very thoroughly before touching the face. Cover cuts and open wounds of the receiver. For FOOT FUNGUS, the receiver must wear clean socks. For FUNGUS ON OTHER AREAS, cover with a clean towel. Change the mat sheets after the session and wash in hot water. Proceed with gentle care.

9. For VASCULAR PROBLEMS, (varicose veins, thrombus, embolus, etc.) Ask receiver to seek medical advice. Avoid pressure on blue or red spider veins. Pressure must be extra-light with slower moves. Seek advice unless you have training and experience to deal with this situation.

10. For DIABETICS, do not hold the pulse pressure points for more than five seconds. Pressure and all other moves must be slower and softer on the feet.

11. For MUSCLE INJURIES, ask receiver to seek medical advice. All moves must be slower and softer on the affected area. Extra support of pillows and other bolsters for

support is recommended. Seek advice unless you have training and experience to deal with this situation.

12. For BONE FRACTURES, ask receiver to seek medical advice. Pressure and all other moves must be slower and softer on the affected area. Use of pillows and other bolsters for support is recommended. Seek advice unless you have training and experience to deal with this situation.

13. For SWELLING and INFLAMMATIONS, ask receiver to seek medical advice. Pressure and other moves must be extra gentle and slower on the affected area. Work around the area when necessary. Seek advice unless you have the training and experience to deal with this situation.

14. For ALCOHOL and DRUG INTOXICATION, ask the receiver to seek medical advice and rehabilitative measures. Re-schedule when the receiver is sober.

15. For HAIR PROBLEMS, (lice, dandruff, falling hair, etc), ask receiver to seek medical advice. Head moves must be extra-gentle for situations with FALLING HAIR. Avoid pulling the hair. Cover the heads of receivers with DANDRUFF or LICE. Change the mat sheets after session and wash in hot water.

16. For FEBRILE CONDITIONS (chills, shivers and temperature), ask receiver to seek medical advice. All moves must be slower and softer. Change the mat sheets after the session.

17. For those with PARKINSON'S CONDITIONS, ask client to seek medical advice. All moves must be firm but slow. Extra support of pillows and bolsters is encouraged during tremors.

18. For those who have been SEXUALLY ABUSED, ask receiver to seek professional counseling. All moves must be very gentle and slower. Provide extra sensitivity and respect for privacy. Use of pillows and other bolsters for support is recommended. Seek advice unless you have the training and experience to deal with this situation.

19. For BACK PROBLEMS, ask receiver to seek medical advice. All moves must be extra-slow and gentle, particularly moves that raise the legs or back, or put pressure on the back or abdomen. Use pillows and bolsters for extra support on the knees, back and abdomen.

20. For those with MEDICAL PORTS (PICC line, hemodialysis catheters, etc.), ask receiver to seek medical advice. Work around the ports. Take extra care to not touch or pull the port. Seek advice unless you have the training experience to deal with this situation.

21. FOR ALL RECEIVERS, a general medical history is a must. Encourage the receiver to express any medical and physical concerns before, during and after the session. Ask permission from the receiver for you to make a follow-up assessment over the phone.

22. When it doubt, leave it out.

Indigenous Advice   Katutubong Payo

    1. Drink water and empty your bladder before and after the session. Water has both yin and yang qualities that prepare the body to yield to the flow and changes that will take place all throughout the process. There is more water in the human body and Mother Earth than anything else. It always was, is and will be here. *This reminds me of the word inog. It means circulating, flowing, and swirling. Let us keep that fluidity working by drinking enough water.*

    2. Immediately after the session, do not expose yourself to anything too cold or hot, such as drinks, food, showers or air. The entire session has an immediate effect of lowering the body's temperature, so sudden exposure to cold or hot will leave you more susceptible to unnecessary patterns of disharmony. *This reminds me of sala sa lamig, sala sa init. It means neither cold nor hot. It is somewhat neutral or room temperature. This refers not just to the body or room temperature but also to one's behaviour such as not aggressive, not withdrawn. You are invited to relax.*

    3. Cleanliness is next to Godliness. It is an important responsibility to be physically clean, to slow down with mental chatters and be at ease with emotions. Be like an empty vessel as you experience hilot. *This reminds me of malinis na puso. This means pure heart. Our thoughts, our actions, and our speech are influenced by our hearts.*

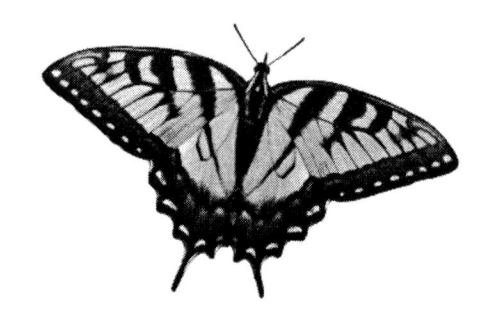

Use Your Body Gamitin ang Iyong Katawan

There are many parts of the giver's body that are used for giving hilot. Knowing how to use parts of the giver's body other than the hands and fingers provide a variety of possibilities for pressure, strength and repositioning necessary for the session.

BALIKAT (SHOULDER)
To support, to anchor, lift and lock, or cover a wide area for pressure, the shoulders are very helpful. Shoulders are protective and have both defensive and offensive energies. They are good to use for leverage for the feet of the receiver and to push against the other person's shoulder, back and hips. The strength of the shoulders determines the strength of the arms and hands.

BISIG (ARM)
Arms for rolling, stretching and support. This is a great technique for areas such as the lateral side of the neck, the back, the limbs, joints such as the knee, hip, lateral side of the lower extremities, and the gluteal fold.

SIKO (ELBOW)
Elbows can be used for support and can give more power for pressure points. The bony structure gives a sharper and deeper pressure that's very useful for massaging the shoulders, lower back and buttocks.

KAMAY (HAND)
Healing hands have a mind of their own. They respond to the first instinct one uses to offer support, nurturing and protection. Use your hands to press, push, grab, grip, sweep, circle, stroke or lock.

KAMAO (FIST)
The fist has an offensive and defensive energy pressure for muscular areas such as the lower back, gluteus, sole of the feet and limbs. Avoid using it on the head, the rib cage, the sternum, the groin, and the joints.

DALIRI sa KAMAY (FINGERS)
To locate pressure points for deeper healing, use your fingers. Some areas, such as the armpit, throat, groins, limbs, spine and internal organs, are more sensitive

The Healing Dance

to the fingers. Be gentle when you use the fingers since they have the ability to find the pain-inducing areas. Only proper touching relieves pain.

LIKOD (BACK)
The back can be a good support for the receiver's back while on a sitting position. It can be used to do wide circles on the trochanter area (near the hip) while the giver's back is slightly bent backward as the receiver lies on the side position.

PUWIT (BUTTOCKS)
To sit on the receiver's gluteal area, inner thigh, and trochanter area is very comfortable for both the giver and receiver. Instantly, it gives an even pressure that covers a wider space.

TUHOD (KNEE)
The knee is for support, for grounding, for a base, for balance, for coordination, for positioning and for massaging pressure points. The giver needs healthy knees to work on the floor a lot. As you kneel, you pray for assistance, humility and surrender. The knee is both an offensive and defensive tool.

PAA (FEET)
Our feet work very hard for us. In everything that we do, they're with us. They carry all our emotions and all our journeys. They are powerful and versatile, making our footwork so much fun. We can use them for balance, positioning, coordination, locking, stretching and pressure. For fun and healing, my son and I like to do a foot fight that brings me somewhat closer to the art of Filipino wrestling. Feet have both defensive and offensive energies. Let your feet roll gently and don't step on the spine and joints. Feet are great for massaging the back and muscular limbs. When you become good at it, you can transform your feet into a snake, a buffalo, a frog, etc. Play with it during the session.

DALIRI sa PAA (TOES)
The toes can be used for massaging pressure points, for hooking and gripping. The pressure they deliver can be stronger than the fingers.

Basic Dance & Weave   Pangunahing Sayaw at Habi

    Filipino hilot is a slow dance, weaving the giver and the receiver to the rhythm of the heart and creating a sacred dance of life. The slow tempo of the dance allows you to modulate your touch in such a way that one touch is able to send and receive a message of healing to a given part of the body, primarily through the body's neural pathways. The silence and the pauses in between the moves allow call-and-response moments and integration of messages between synapses in the body that lead the dancers and weavers. There is a kinetic vibration that radiates to make the necessary changes in energy beyond what we can touch to the unseen bodies of the mind and the heart. The body resists less at a slow tempo. When there is less resistance, the energy wave flows more freely. Thus, one can restore and achieve patterns of harmony.

    Time and space for each motion are well-received by the body. Each cell is given adequate time and space to communicate with others, to study the steps together and get ready for the next move. The slow tempo also allows the body to thoroughly digest, assimilate and absorb each step. Every move is like a switch in gears. Each change of gear leads to a much-needed shifting of the body part. When there's a shift, there's a change in the vibrational flow.

    Although some of the movements listed below are also observed in other forms of indigenous massage, it is in Thai massage that I have experienced all of them in one session. It is not only the fact that all motions can be experienced in this indigenous massage, but the beauty of it is the order and pattern of the dance that is woven is in order and harmony with the diwatas and the universe.

    As you dance and weave through hilot, a pattern of togetherness is formed. Two people with close physical contact support each other for growth just like bamboo plants that grow taller, greener, stronger and in abundance. Being together, support is generated. I have listed the movements according to the frequency of use, from the most frequently used to the least. Each motion, whether most used or least used, contributes to the completion of the dance and weave.

    Practice unceasingly so as to make each movement free of conscious thought. Halina't magsayaw (Let's dance!)

PAGHINGA (BREATH)
Take a deep breath. Inhale and exhale deeply and slowly through your nose. Notice the cool air as you inhale and warm air as you exhale. Do this three times. Your abdomen inflates as you inhale and deflates as you exhale. There is harmony as the giver and receiver synchronize each other's breathing with the motions. Inhale healing energy and visualize the colors of the rainbow through your chakras and bring all joy, love, peace, courage, faith, trust and acceptance. Exhale to let go of all the discomforts, worries, problems, complaints, confusions, conflicts, burdens, doubts, fears, aches and pains. Through breath comes life and transformation. There is space when you inhale and exhale that makes an impact on our mindfulness to ourselves and others.

PISIL o DIIN (SQUEEZE or PRESS)
The receiver's entire body, except for the genital area, is pressed by the giver's hands, fingers, feet, forearm, elbows, knees, back and buttocks. Presses are good for warming up the body for the next move. Using different parts of the body allows different energy levels for both the giver and the receiver. It is also a way for the giver to not overuse one part of the body.

HELE (ROCK)
Rock as you press. Rock when you stretch. Rock from side to side. Rock forward and backward. Rocking keeps the slow rhythm that allows adequate time for each cell to respond to the movement with good blood circulation that provides oxygen, nutrients and antibodies, and releases toxins from the body. To rock is to comfort, to support and to nurture. It lulls both dancers to a calm and quiet time and space. It is a portrait of diwata nurturing her child.

PABILOG (CIRCLE)
Circles can be done with the palm, fingers (particularly the thumb), foot, heels and big toe. They are soothing to use at the beginning and at the end of a deep pressure.

BALUKTOT at IKOT (BEND and ROTATE)
The saying, "A chain is only as strong as its weakest link," is not only true to a chain, but to the human body as well. Our joints are our links. Joints are structured heavily. Cartilages, fasciae, nerves, blood vessels, connective tissues and lymph glands meet to form bridges that allow the body to function systematically. If not bent and rotated, congestion can occur, slowing down or occluding the normal flow of energy. To bend and rotate enhances lubrication of fluids and opens up the pathways for necessary nutrients, enzymes and antibodies.

In a dance, bending and rotation give a dramatic effect that adds beauty and magic to the whole dance. It is important to pay attention to even the smallest joint. Each joint, no matter how small, contributes to health of all other joints.

INAT (STRETCH)
To stretch is to elongate, to reach out and to make the body and mind more flexible. When flexibility is attained, we are better able to tolerate and endure aches, pains and other discomforts. We also make more room for loving kindness and compassion to oneself and others. Our mind and body becomes pliant like the bamboo that bends in all directions with the wind. And like the bamboo plant we can reach out to provide nourishment, shelter, protection and support.

KAPIT (HOOK)
Hooking provides additional support, pressure and stretching. Use your fingers and toes to hook the shoulder blade, gluteal fold, legs and upper arms. An example would be, as the receiver lay on the back and the giver sits next to the receiver's shoulder being worked on, the giver's toes are hooked into the shoulder blade while fingers are hooked into the shoulder creating a pull-and-push effect. Another example would be for the giver's toes to hook the gluteal fold of the receiver as the giver stretches the leg being hooked towards the giver.

TAPIK at TADTAD (CUP and CHOP)
The body is a human drum and drumming brings out the rhythm of one's soul in harmony with diwata and the universe. The sound and vibration when you chop and cup the muscular and areas of the body, such as the legs, back, upper arms, shoulder, chest and neck, resonates healing waves that travels beyond the confines of our physical bodies. It is a powerful way to communicate with the diwata, ninuno, loved ones and all beings. The rhythm drives away unnecessary negativities, helps release energetic blockages, promotes circulation, relaxes body, mind and spirit, and invites the spaciousness needed to process our growth and healing. It is like music to the ears and whole body. Avoid this motion on the spine areas of the neck and back.

LAMAS (KNEAD)
Kneading the muscular areas such as the arms and legs softens and smoothes the muscles, getting rid of uncomfortable knots. When muscles are smooth, change takes place in a more flowing manner. Knots cause congestion that alters the smooth flow conducive for healing.

GULONG at PADULAS (ROLL and SLIDE)
Rolling and sliding are executed using the forearms. Rolling is especially good for massaging the neck, pelvis and sacral area, while the receiver is on the side, back

or in a sitting position. It provides a good feeling of continuity of touch with no interruption. It is a good way to convey the message, "I am here for you."

HAPLOS (SWEEP)

There is more to our bodies than our physical bodies. To sweep is to work on the energy field on the outer body. In our traditions, we always hear grandparents reminding us to be careful when we are sweeping our homes, particularly at night since we might sweep and disrespect forces in nature living with us. When a child suddenly gets sick, parents have to recall the strangers to whom the child has been exposed recently who might have caused the discomfort due to the stranger's energy. That stranger has to come to the child's rescue by placing and sweeping one's hands on the abdominal area, at the bottom of the feet and on top of the head to get rid of whatever is bothering the child. This is believed to be true since outer bodies are meant to protect and nurture the physical bodies. When the giver sweeps the receiver, the intention is to clean out unwanted toxins and negativities that do not contribute to the harmony of the receiver's mind, body, heart and spirit.

ANGAT at HILA (LIFT and PULL)

To lift and to pull, balances the constant force of gravity weighing the body down. It allows the body to be elevated and yet be grounded all at the same time. It creates equilibrium in our being. When the giver uses her arms to balances and positions herself and the receiver puts his trust in the giver, it conveys a message of, "No matter how heavy your heart is, it will be lifted, elevated and released as long as you trust, accept, surrender and let go. Nothing is too heavy."

SARA (LOCK)

To lock with the limbs in combination with a hook or press allows another angle of pressure and balance. Coordination, flexibility and balance are needed to execute this move.

PIHIT (PIVOT)

This is a subtle but powerful motion. As the giver holds the receiver's feet and hands, balancing with one foot on the ground and the other foot on the receiver's back, the giver executes a tiny, yet delightful, twist of the hips and lower back further, working on chakras 1 and 2. Even a small motion like this is considered significant and important. It is not how big or strong the motion is. It has a special place in the healing dance and weave. Anything and everything is medicine.

PILIPIT (TWIST)
This is done gently and slowly with both hands doing a slight rotation on two opposite directions, upper hand goes counter clockwise and lower hand goes clockwise. This is another way to loosen entangled tissues, muscles, nerves and fasciae. There are times when we feel overwhelmed, distraught, confused, achy or tight because our bodies, thoughts, emotions, words, and actions may be twisted, misaligned or cluttered. To untwist releases and lets go of these uncomfortable possibilities, allow us to relax and provides space for diwata to do its work with us.

These motions are not the only ones that you can do. You are invited to explore your own patterns of creativity and imagination. These motions of dance and weaving condition our ways of knowing, thinking and being for serendipity, synchronicity and harmony.

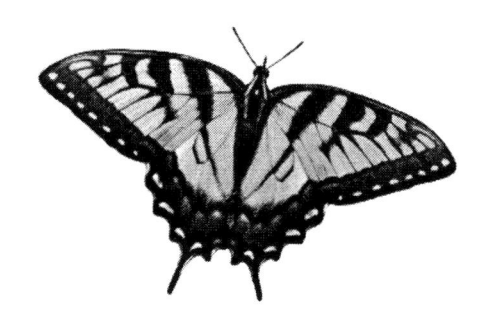

INTRODUCTION TO TRADITIONAL THAI MASSAGE

In the illustrations, broken arrows designate alternate palm presses, finger presses or rocking motions.

I. FRONT POSITION

First Chakra — Numbers 1-9

1. CLEANSING, GROUNDING AND CENTERING

a. The giver's hands and feet must be clean.

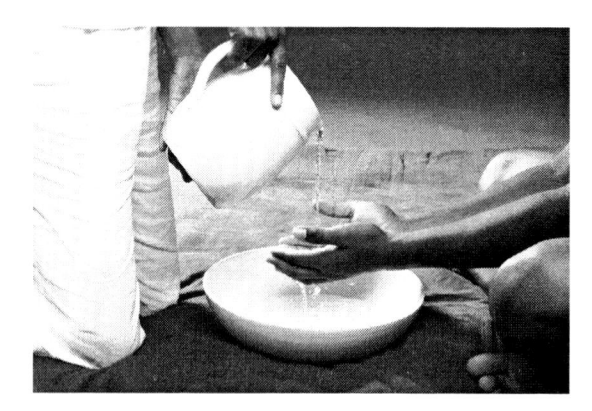

1 (a) Life is water

b. The giver cleans the receiver's feet with a warm wash cloth. Alternatively, the receiver's feet must be soaked in warm water with sea salt and an essential oil or herbal infusion.

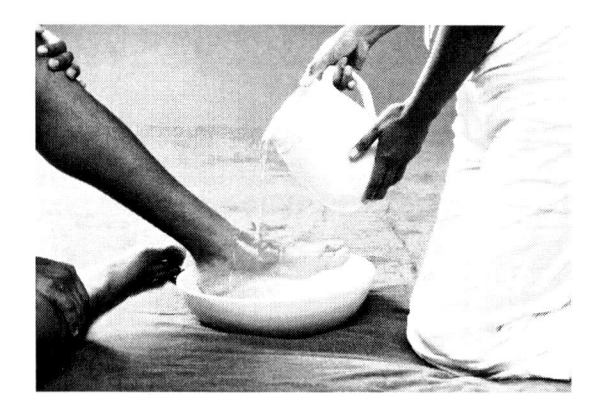

1 (b) We are water and we are life

c. The giver and receiver begin with three cleansing breaths. Inhale through the nose and exhale through the mouth.

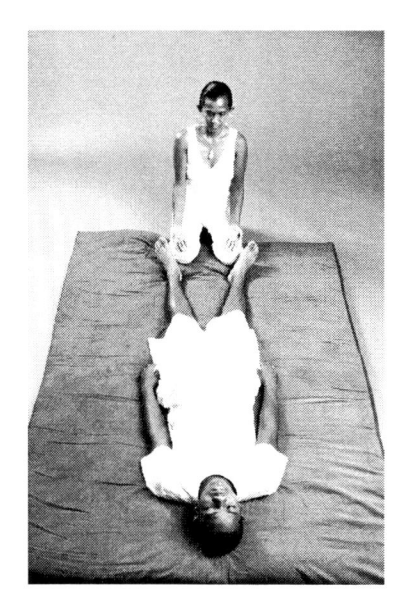

1 (c) Healing mantra

2. OM NAMO PERSONAL PRAYER AND MEDITATION

a. At the beginning of each session, start with OM NAMO or any prayer for healing, peace, thanksgiving and guidance for both the giver and receiver. Call upon the Creator and the ancestral spirits.

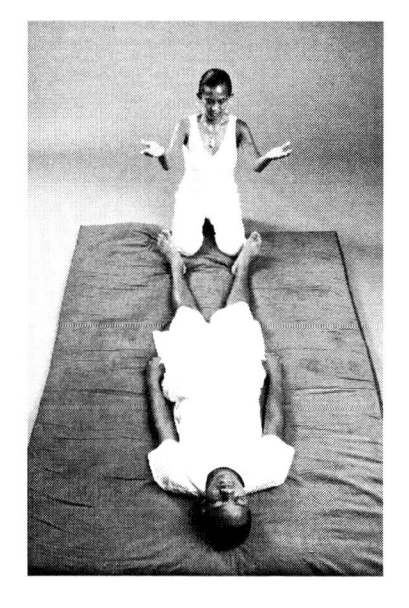

2 (a) Pray for healing

3. WARMING THE GIVER'S HANDS AND HEART

a. Receiver lies on the back with hands at the sides and breathing normally. The giver puts her hands together near the heart and rubs hands together until warm.

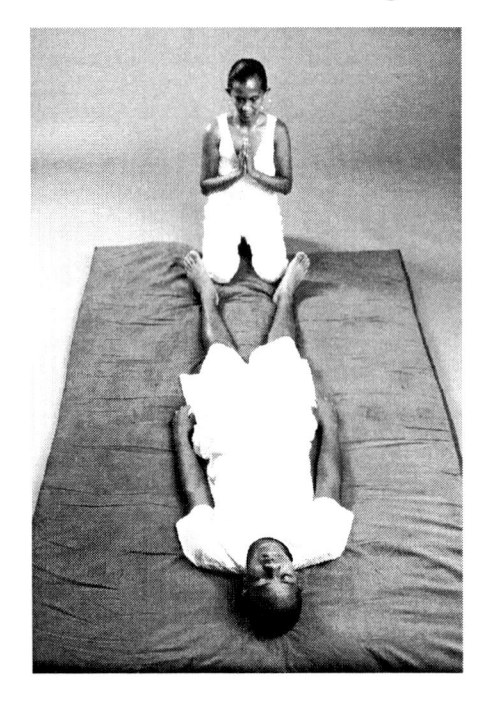

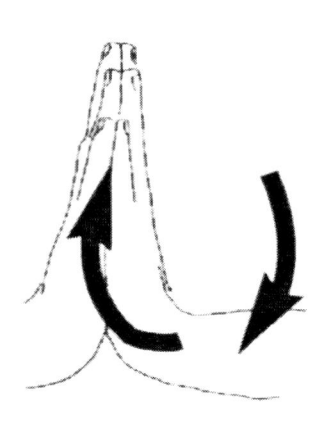

3 (a) Pray for healing

b. Be in tune with the receiver's breathing. On exhalation, rock forward and backward as you softly and gently palm-press the feet together.
(Three times)

4. SAY HELLO TO THE FEET

Starting on the feet is less invasive when doing massage. It is also a good way to do an initial assessment of the receiver's tension and flexibility. It also opens up the energy lines.

a. Place your hands gently on the receiver's bilateral medial arch.

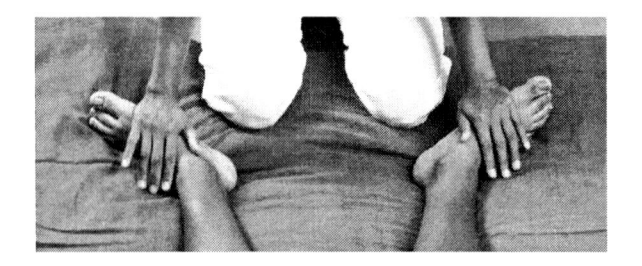

36 *Grace Sunga Asagra*

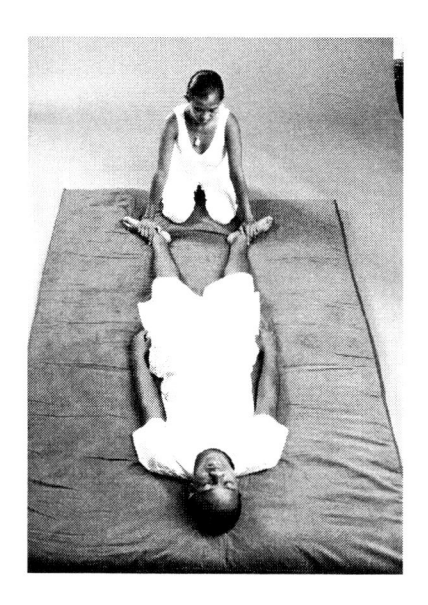

4 (a) Searching for the roots

b. Notice the receiver's breathing and be in tune with it. As the receiver exhales, gently palm-press together the feet and rock from side to side. Do this three times.

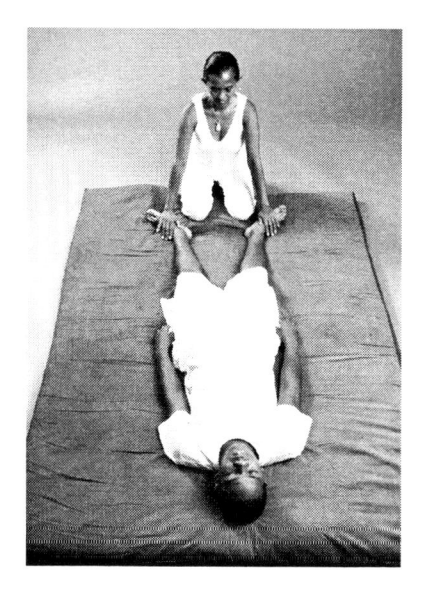

4 (b) Heating bamboo

5. ROCKING

a. The giver rocks side to side and alternately palm-presses the receiver's feet, moving from the ankles to medial arch to the toes, then back to the medial arch and to the ankles.

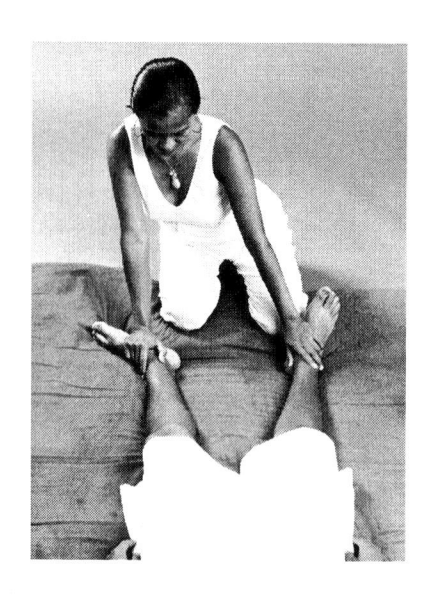

5 (a) Heating bamboo

6. ELEPHANT WALKING

a. Imagine you're an elephant.

With your hands, walk with strength, power, confidence, assurance and grace by rocking and alternately pressing up the medial sides of the legs.
(Three alternating presses each side)

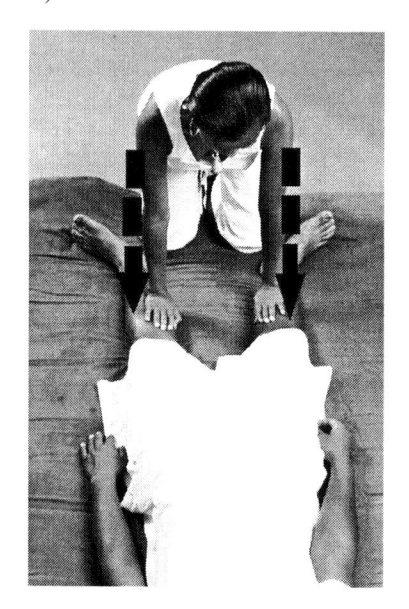

6 (a) Heating bamboo

b) Gently palm circle both knees in an outward motion (left hand counter-clockwise and right hand – clockwise). Pay extra careful attention to the patella.

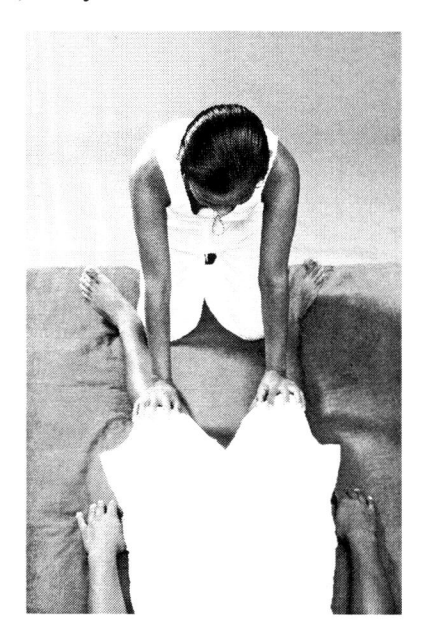

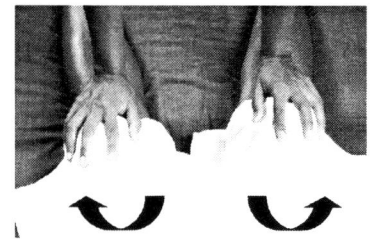

6 (b) Heating bamboo

c. Proceed with alternate palm from the quadriceps to the pulses (three presses on each side). The giver's fingers are spread and towards the head.

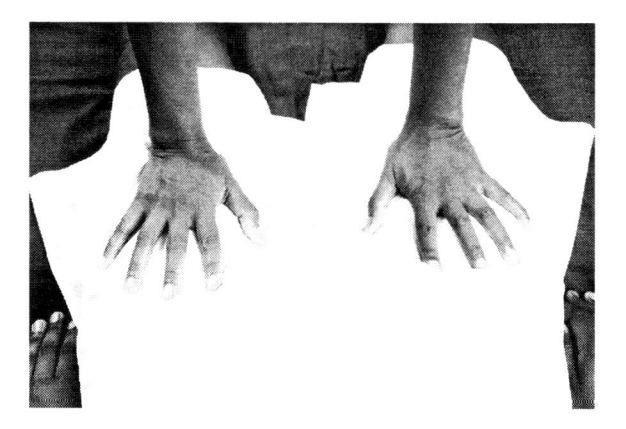

6 (c) Rocking the gate

d. Keep your hands together and pause. Hold the pulse for one second on the bilateral femoral pulse points.

The Healing Dance   39

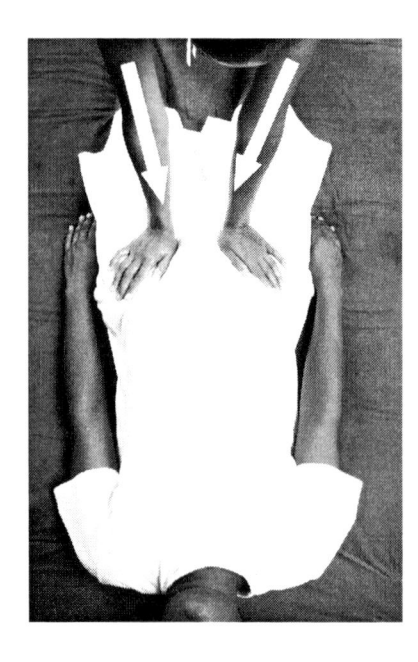

6 (d) Rocking the gate

e. Release the pressure. Keep your hands together over the energy field of the pulses for a second, then proceed to the next step.

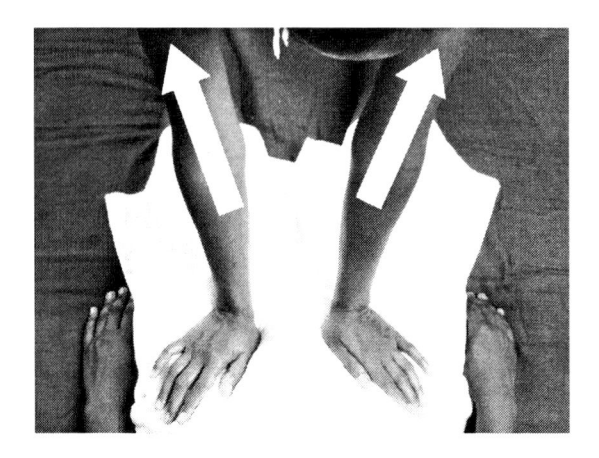

6 (e) Opening the gate

f. Gently alternate palm-presses all the way down to the ankles. Maintain the same slow rhythm and distances from the femoral pulses to the knees then to the ankles.

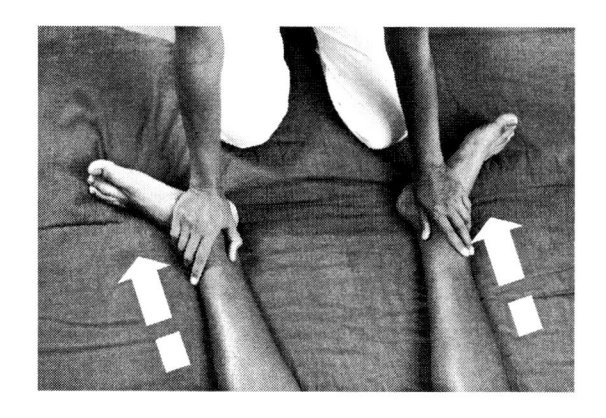

6 (f) Heating bamboo

7. SIX POINTS

a. Palm-press from ankles (soft) to middle of the feet (hard) to the toes (soft.)

b. Rock forward and backward as you thumb press the six points with the order as follows:

> SOFT pressure on points 1 for 5 seconds.
> SOFT pressure on points 2 for 5 seconds.
> SOFT pressure on points 3 for 5 seconds.
> SOFT pressure on points 4 for 5 seconds.
> SOFT pressure on points 5 for 5 seconds.
> SOFT pressure on points 6 for 5 seconds.

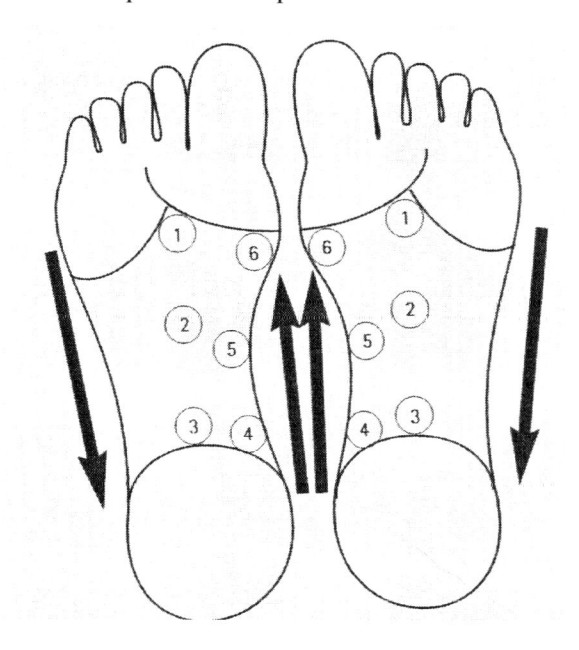

Then go back to points one and repeat the cycle increasing pressure from SOFT to HARD to SOFT.
(A total of three cycles)

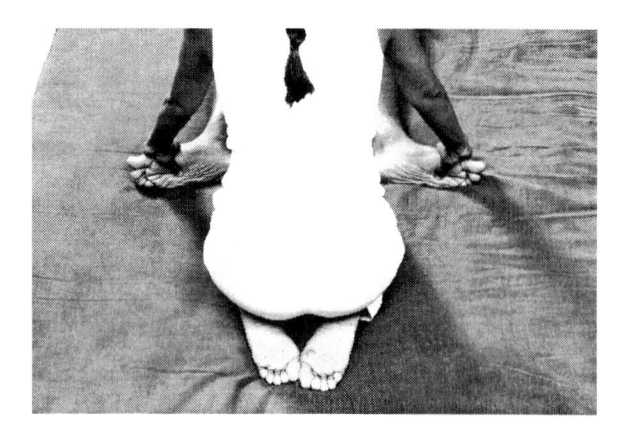

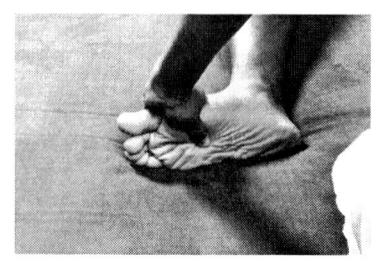

7 (b) Stimulate yin and yang

c. Close the trails with a gentle alternate rocking and alternate palm-presses on the feet.

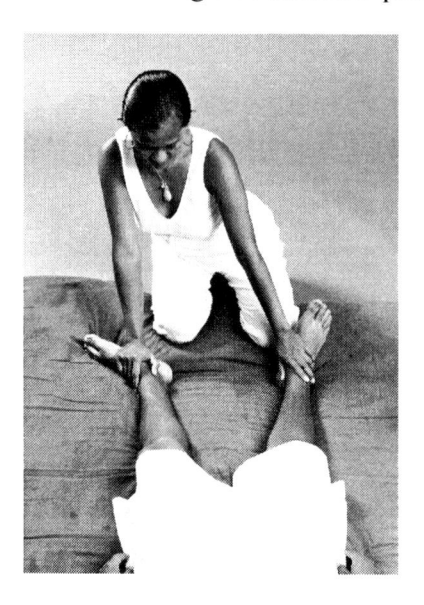

7 (c) Stimulate yin and yang

8. FIVE TRAILS (BOTTOM OF THE FEET)

a. Hold both feet together. Rock forward and backward as you thumb-press the trails on the soles of the feet, starting with POINT 3 (in front of the heel), down each little trail that leads to the ball of each toe, where you change from thumb-presses to thumb circles. START WITH THE BIG TOE (trail 1) until you end up with the little toe (trail 5).

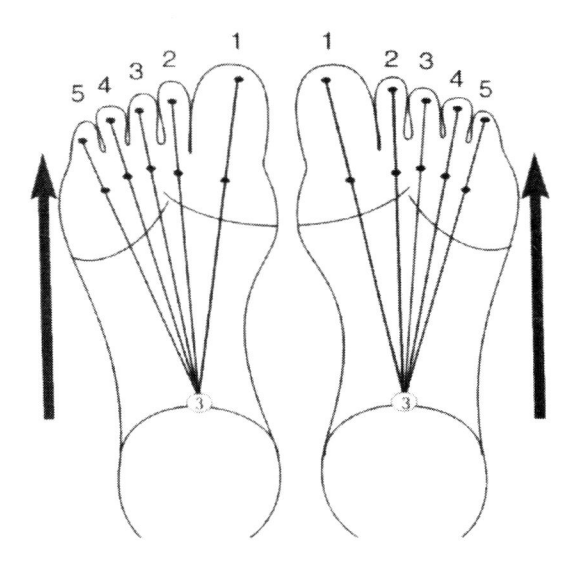

Approximately four presses from point 3 to the ball of each toe. Thumb circles at the ball of each toe.

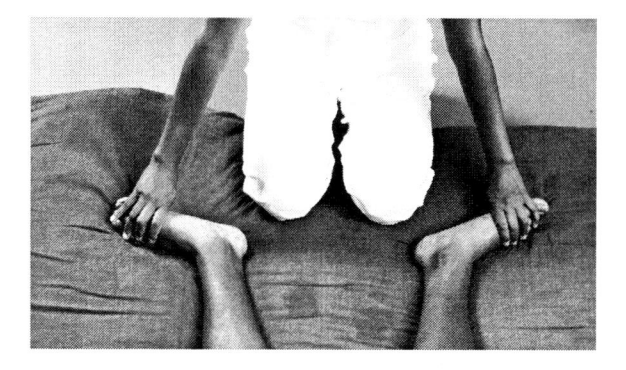

8 (a) Stimulate yin and yang

b. End with a gentle SQUEEZE, PINCH and gentle SNAP of each toe.

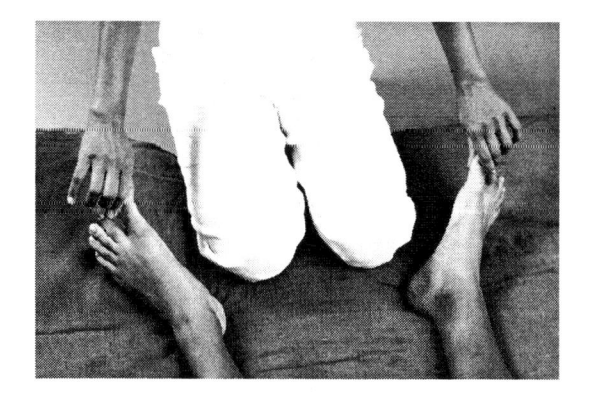

8 (b) Maiden picks flower buds

The Healing Dance 43

c. Close the trails with a gentle alternate rocking and alternate palm-presses of the feet.

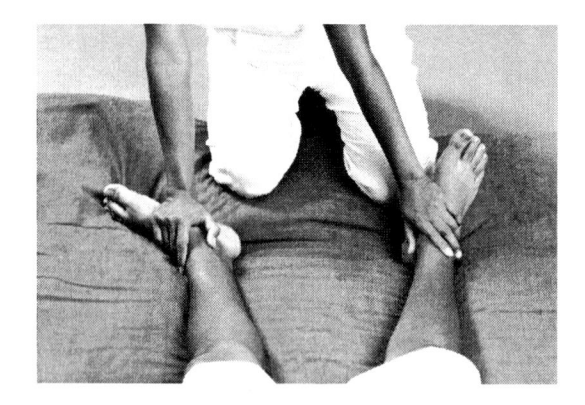

8 (c) Stimulate yin and yang

9. FOUR CANALS (TOP OF THE FEET)

a. Hold the feet together to pave the way to the canals by rocking and pressing together in front of the ankle, the middle of the foot over the arch, and the toes. (Three simultaneous palm-presses from ankles to mid-foot to toes — soft-hard-soft)

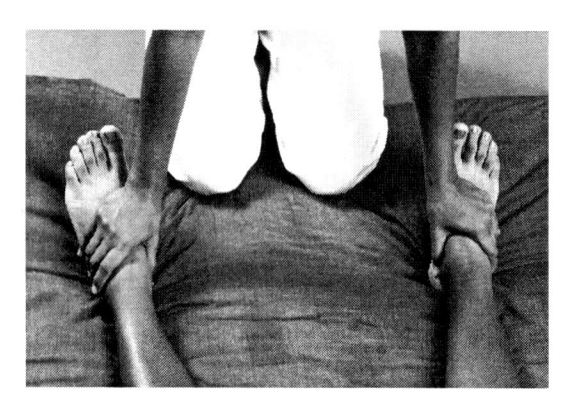

9 (a) Seizing bamboo

b. Rock forward and press together the depression at the top of the ankle (St 41) followed by thumb circles on the grooves, all the way to each TOE WEB STARTING FROM THE BIG TOE (canal one). First groove is found between the big toe and the second toe. Second groove is between the second and third toe, and so on. For the fifth toe, with the giver's middle finger, thumb circle along the side of the foot. Always go back to the depression as you thumb circle each canal to each web.

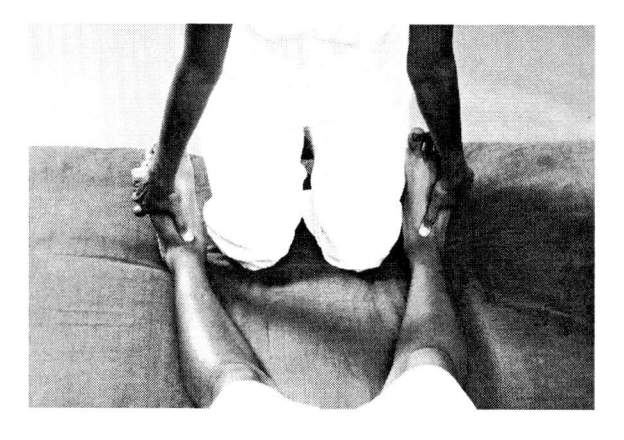

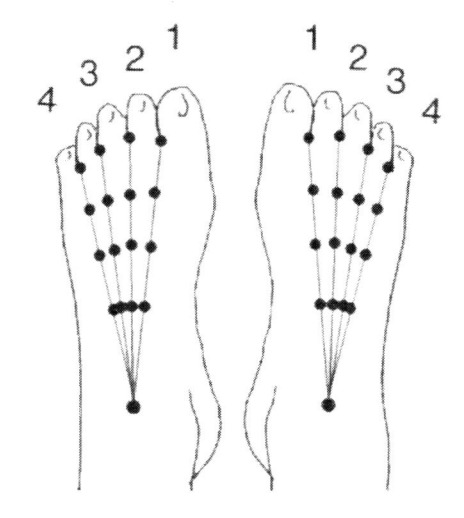

9 (b) Cracking bamboo

c. At the end of each toe, slip off with a SQUEEZE AND PULL.

Cracking may or may not be heard. If heard, finish the cracking toe with a thumb circle on top of the knuckle.

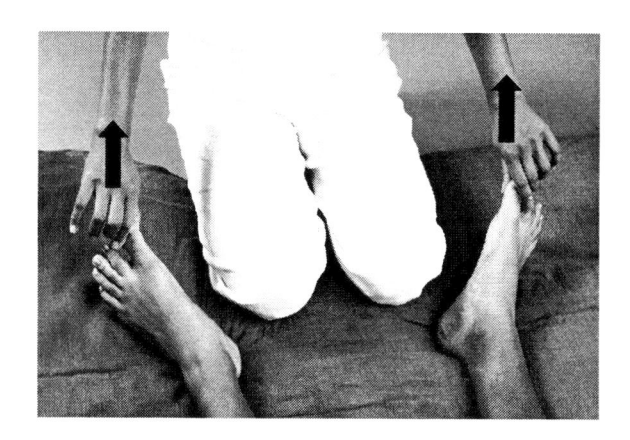

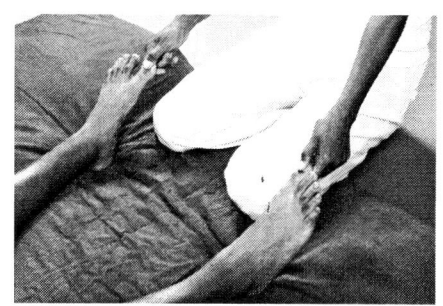

9 (c) Maiden picks flower buds

10. ROTATE ANKLES:

First and Fifth Chakras

Each ankle will be rotated one at a time.
For a woman, start with the left ankle.
For a man, start with the right ankle.

a. Face the receiver, hold the foot of choice, sit down at an angle diagonal to the foot of choice.
Female Receiver

The Healing Dance 45

The heel of the giver's right hand rests on the ball of the receiver's right foot while the giver's left palm supports the receiver's right heel.

The giver's right leg is extended and gently supported, allowing the receiver's right leg (especially the knee) to rest on the giver's extended right leg.

Follow these directions from the opposite side for male receivers. Begin on the right side.

b. With hands and legs in position as instructed, using the giver's waist as the fulcrum, lean forward and make a counterclockwise, gentle, circular motion of the giver's body while stretching the heels and feet of the receiver.

Five cycles in one direction (counterclockwise), then five cycles in the opposite direction. (clockwise)

Female Receiver:

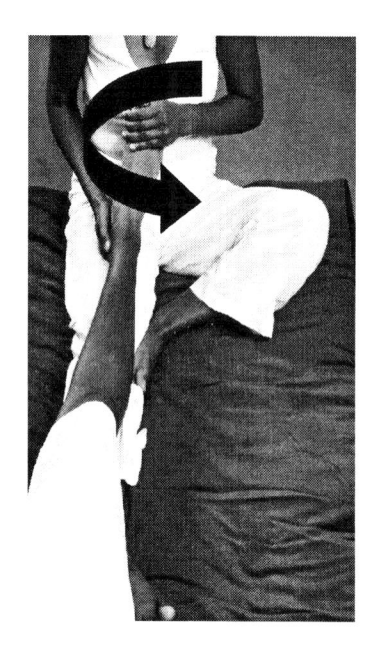

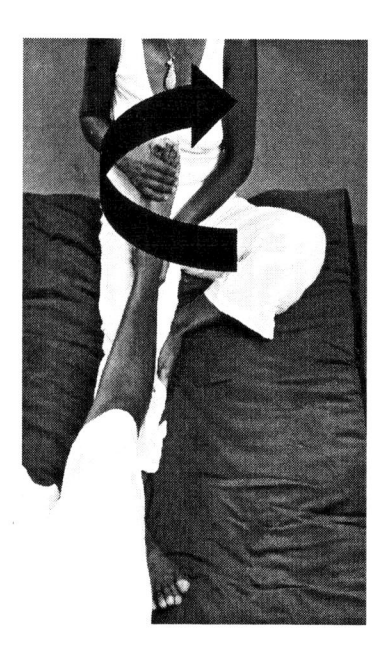

10 (b) Twisting the bamboo

c. The heel of the receiver's left foot rests on the left palm of the giver. The heel of the giver's right hand holds onto the ball of the receiver's left foot. The giver's left leg is extended underneath the receiver's left leg where the knee is resting.

d. Rotate in clockwise motion five times and rotate counterclockwise. (five times)

Your body weight, your hands, your waist and the circular motions must work in harmony to push, stretch and pull the ankle. This powerful movement allows the entire leg-hip structure to loosen all the way up to the side of the neck.

Male Receiver

Start on the right foot of the male receiver and follow the same moves as above.

11. TWIST FOOT:

First Chakra – Numbers 11-14

a. With the heel of the receiver's foot resting on the giver's palm, use the giver's hand to grasp the medial arch and rock back and forth while twisting the foot from the arch to the heels to the toes and back.

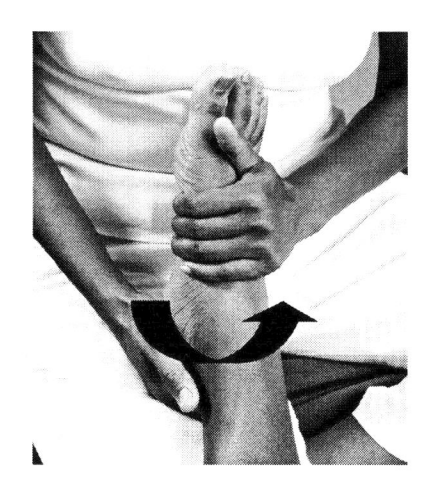

11 (a) Maiden picks flowers

b. Switch hands and repeat the rocking and twisting movement with the lateral side of the foot, opposite the medial arch, to the heels to the toes and back.
(soft-hard-soft-hard-soft)

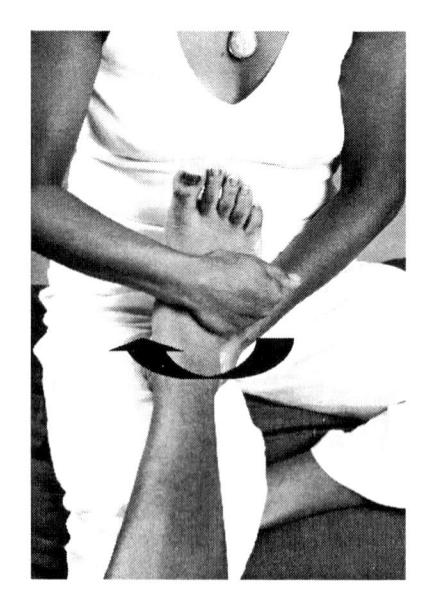

11 (b) Maiden picks flowers

12. PULLING TOES

a. With one hand holding the receiver's heel, hold each toe between the thumb and the index finger.

Begin with the big toe. Loosen and work on the joints of the toes by rotating each toe several times.

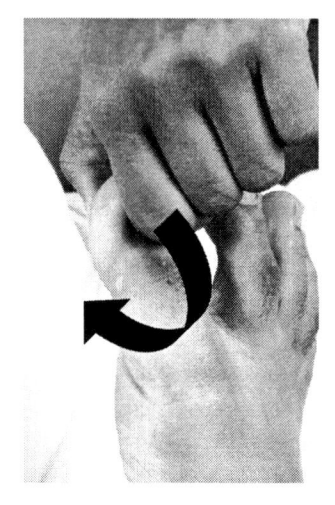

12 (a) Maiden picks flower buds

b. Hold firmly at the base of each toe and pull back as you lean back. You may use the thumb and the index finger to pull.

The toe may or may not make a cracking sound. If it cracks, move on to the next toe.

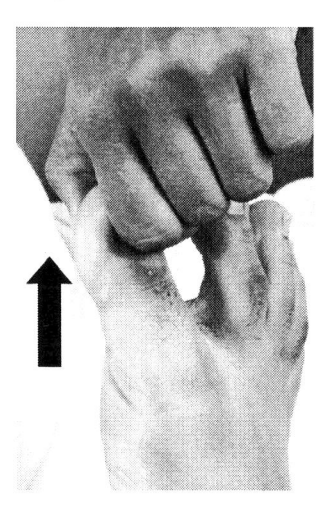

12 (b) Maiden picks flower buds

c. Press and knead the foot with both hands.

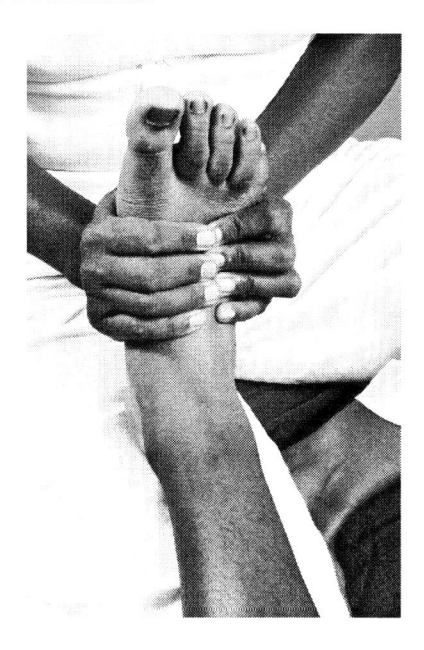

12 (c) Maiden picks flower

13. PLANTAR FLEXION

a. Rock forward and backward as you palm press together the top of the feet, from ankles to toes and back (soft-hard-soft).

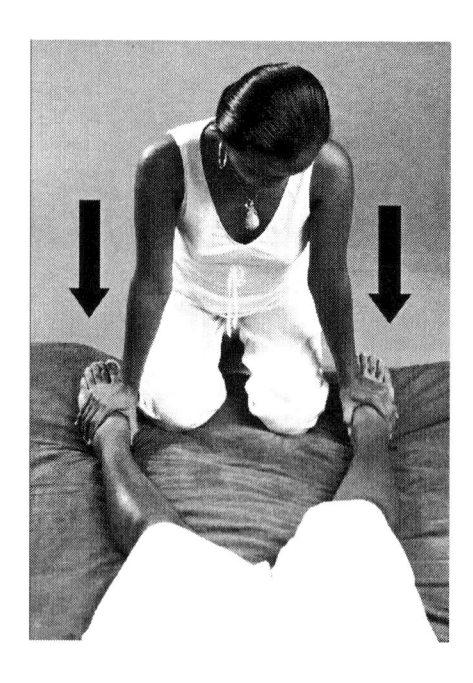

13 (a) Seizing bamboo

14. KNEE UPRIGHT

First Chakra

a. With the receiver's knee in an upright position and the giver kneeling and facing the receiver, the giver secures the receiver's foot by using her knees and thighs. The giver hooks the fingertips of one hand in front of the fingertips of the other hand on the centerline of the receiver's thigh, above the knee. Rock back and forth as you pull into the centerline with the fingertips.

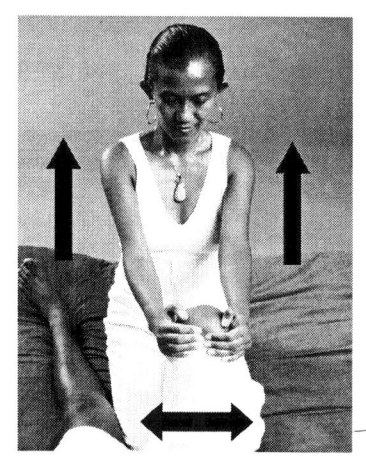

14 (a) Pulling up roots

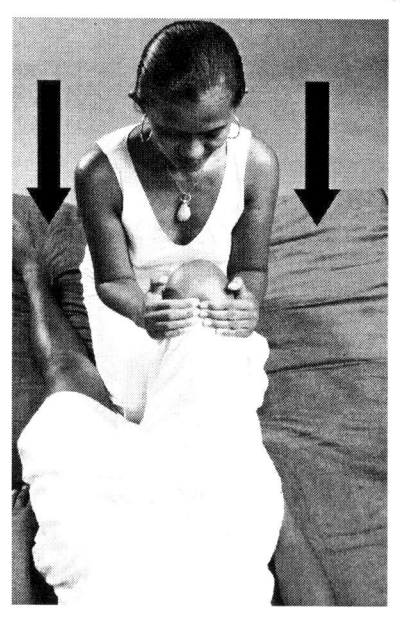

50 *Grace Sunga Asagra*

b. Adjust your hands and fingertips to cover from the knee to mid-thigh to the upper thigh, and back to the knee of the receiver.

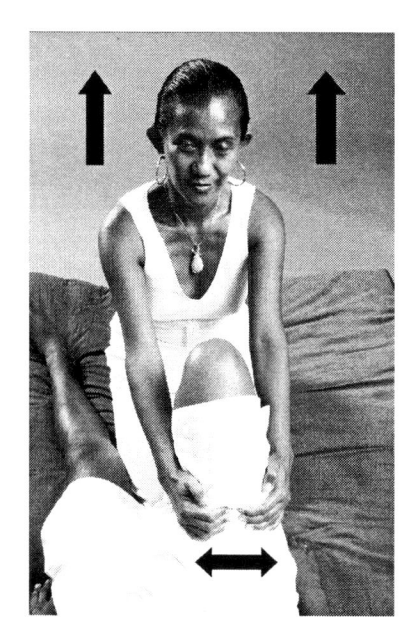

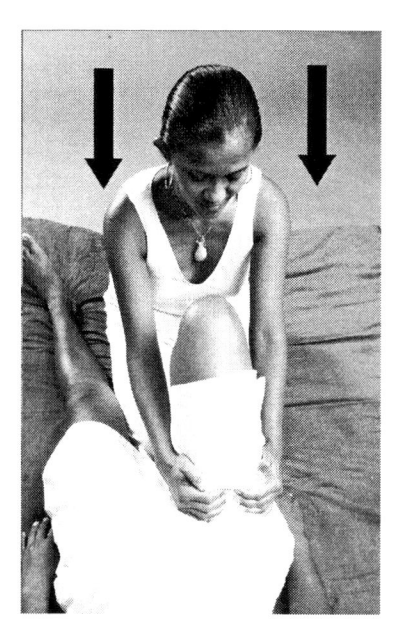

14 (b) Pulling up roots

15. NUTCRACKER

a. Anchor the receiver's foot towards the his buttocks while the giver's buttocks stays as close to the ground as possible.

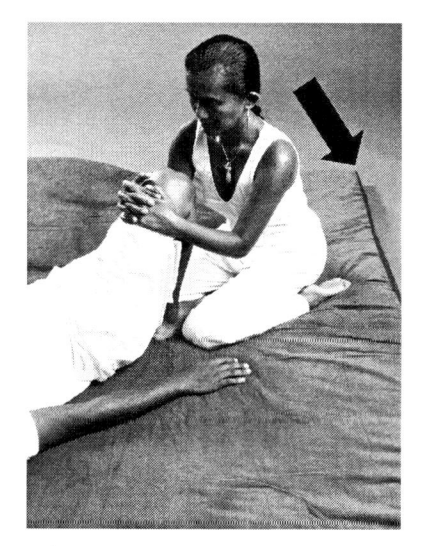

15 (a) Praying mantis catches prey

b. Giver sits as close to the floor as possible.

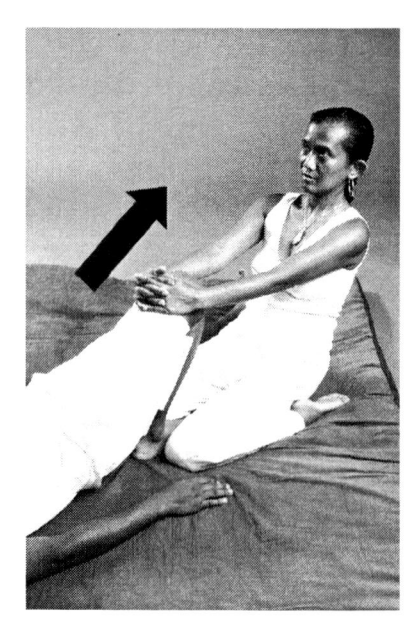

15 (b) Praying mantis catches prey

c. Interlace your fingers and place the heel of the hand against the outside and inside lines starting above the knee. Press and squeeze firmly. Lean back with your body, your head tilted back, and pull. Move from knee to mid-thigh to groin and back. Feel and see the stretch on the receiver's back. This is a favorite stretch of most.

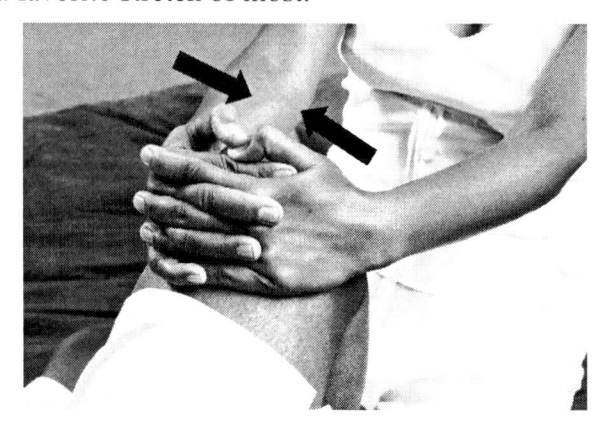

15 (c) Praying mantis catches prey

16. KNEE TO CHEST — ONE HAND

First and Second Chakras (Numbers 15 to 19)

a. The giver, while in a half kneeling stance, faces the receiver. Bend and raise the receiver's leg and anchor the receiver's bent leg on the giver's raised groin (the outside leg) while the other leg (in a kneeling position) supports the receiver's straight leg on the medial side. If the receiver is tall and flexible, the receiver has to adjust the stance closer to the receiver's shoulder. With the giver's hands supporting the receiver's raised and bent knee, do some gentle circular movements of the leg. Do these five times clockwise and then reverse.

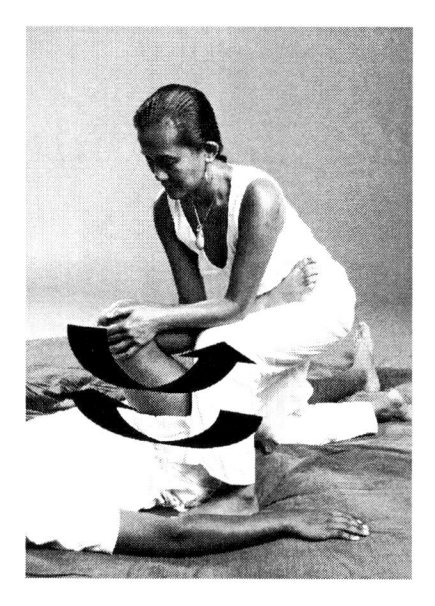

16 (a) Unlock chi

b. With the giver's inside hand on the upper thigh just below the groin and the outside hand, steadily support the receiver's raised knee while rocking forward and back three times — soft-hard-soft. With the other hand on the straight leg, palm-press gently from upper to mid-thigh to just above the knee and then back.

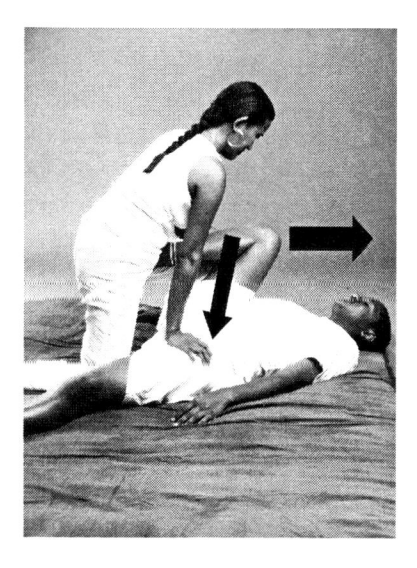

16 (b) Unlock chi

c. If the receiver's straight leg becomes unsteady, the giver can place one's foot across the receiver's straight leg particularly on the receiver's ankle

17. KNEE TO CHEST—TWO HANDS—
BUTTERFLY HAND:

a. Continue on a half–kneeling stance with both hands on the back of the thigh with heels of the hands side by side looking like a butterfly. Rock forward as the giver pushes with hands from the knee to mid-thigh to upper thigh.

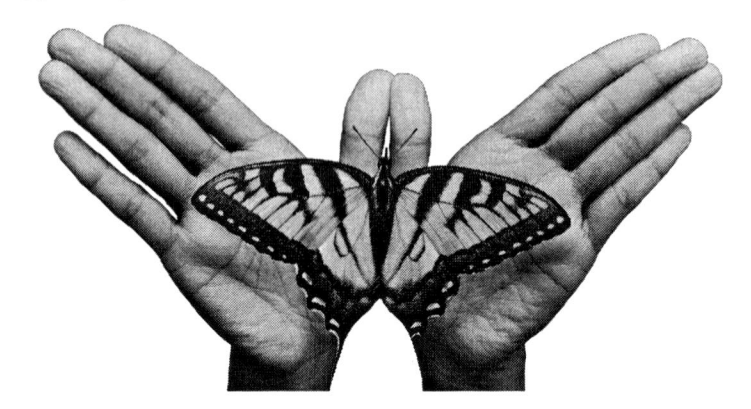

18. DROP KNEE—ONE HAND PRESS

a. Drop the receiver's knee outward, supporting it with your outside hand. Rock downward as the inside hand palm-presses from knee to mid-thigh to groin (soft–hard-soft) and then back to mid-thigh to groin.

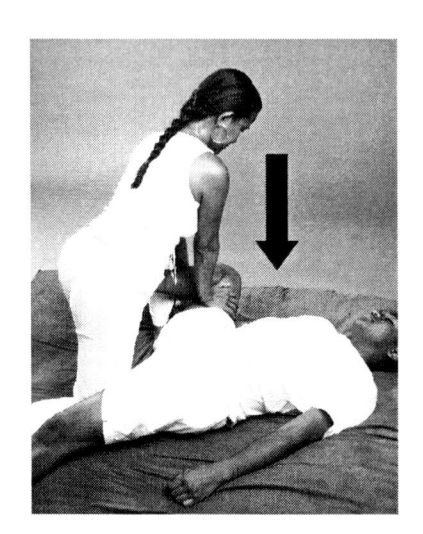

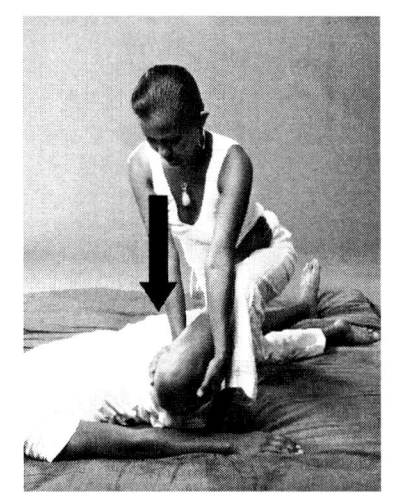

18 (a) Unlock chi

54 *Grace Sunga Asagra*

19. ROCKING THE HIPS

a. The giver maintains a half-kneeling stance while the receiver's knee remains in an upright position. This time the raised leg of the giver is on the opposite side of the raised knee of the receiver. The giver gently guides the foot of her bent leg across the receiver's straight leg. Place your outside foot beside the lateral area of the receiver's bent foot. The hand that is on the side of your raised leg supporting the receiver's foot will be on the receiver's raised knee; your other hand on the receiver hip. Alternately rocks and palm-press the knee and hips (three to five cycles), increasing in pressure gently and gradually.

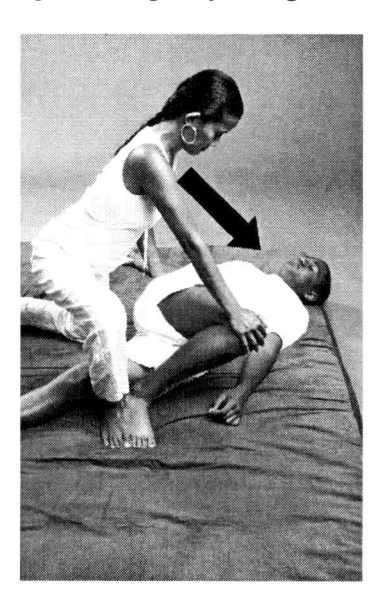

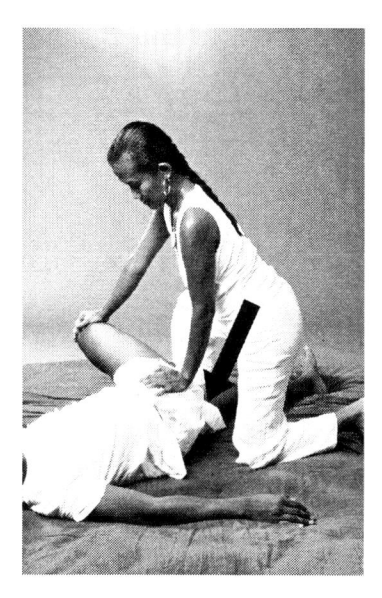

19 (a) Unlock chi

b. To end, guide the bent leg with one hand on the knee and the other hand on the ankle to straighten it up. Shake it and lie it gently beside the straight leg.

c. Now you are ready to repeat the process with the other leg and do the "dance step," starting with the knee upright.

20. ABDOMINAL CARE: THE HARA

First, Second and Third Chakras

a. The receiver lies comfortably on the back with a small pillow support his knee. The giver sits or kneels on the right side of the receiver and gently places the hand over the navel for a few breaths.

The Healing Dance

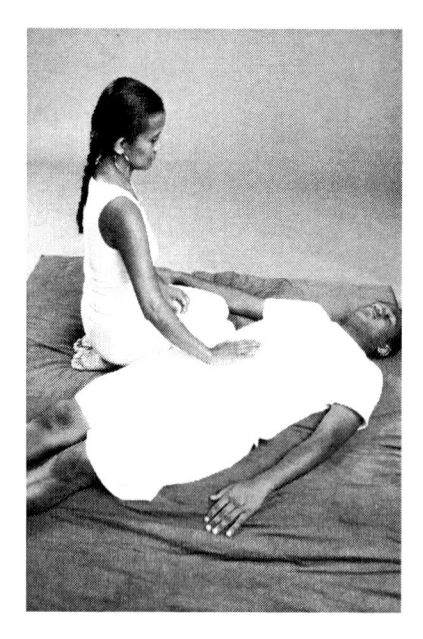

20 (a) Mixing the cauldron of the five elements

b. Proceed with palm circles in a clockwise motion, imagining a ripple effect so the circle starts from the navel and gets bigger, extending to the entire perimeters of the abdomen (below the ribs and above the pubic bone).

RIPPLE-LIKE CIRCLES. (five to seven circles depending on the size of the person.)

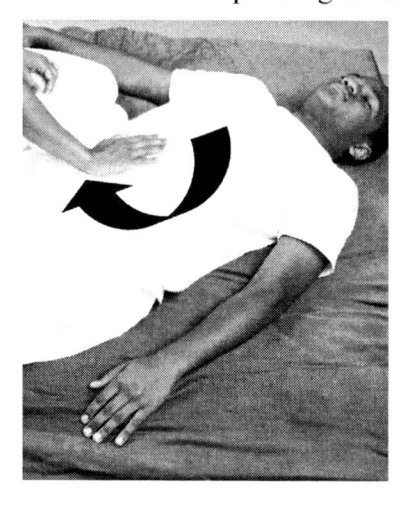

20 (b) Mixing the cauldron of the five elements

c. Make small circles starting from the first point to the ninth point all over the abdomen. This allows the giver to become sensitive to the situation of the hara. Different areas of the hands (whole palm, heel of palm, and flat part of the fingers) can be used to feel the entire abdomen.

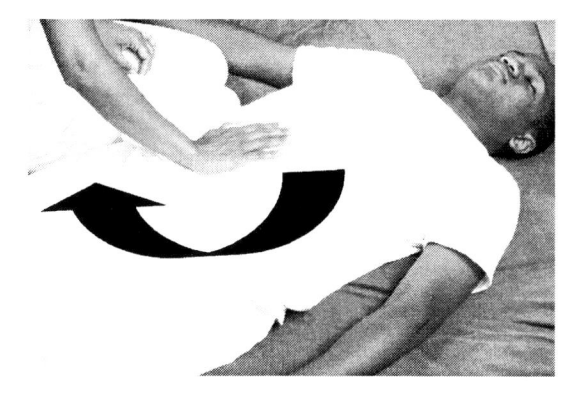

20 (c) Mixing the cauldron of the five elements

d. Gently rest the palm over the navel for a few breaths.

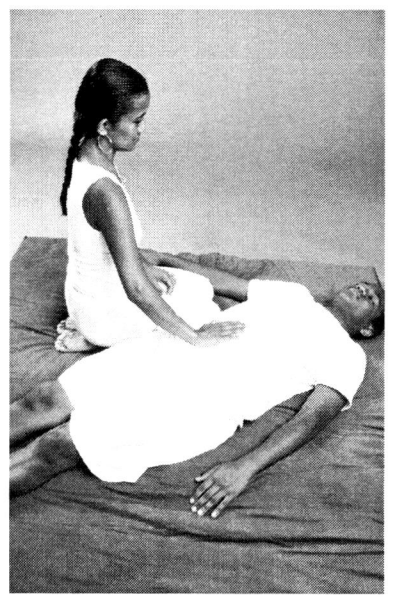

20 (d) Mixing the cauldron of the five elements

Get ready to do the nine points.
The location of the nine points are as follows:

1. right of center of the pubic bone, somewhere at 6:30 on a clock.
2. at the pelvic rim, at 8:00
3. at the waist, at 9:00
4. at the bottom of the ribs on the right side, between 10:30 and 11:30
5. below the sternum at 12:00, at the bottom of the ribs on the left side,
6. between points 5 and 7, at 1:30
7. at the waist, 3:00

The Healing Dance 57

8. at the pelvic rim, 4:30
9. parallel to point one, 5:30

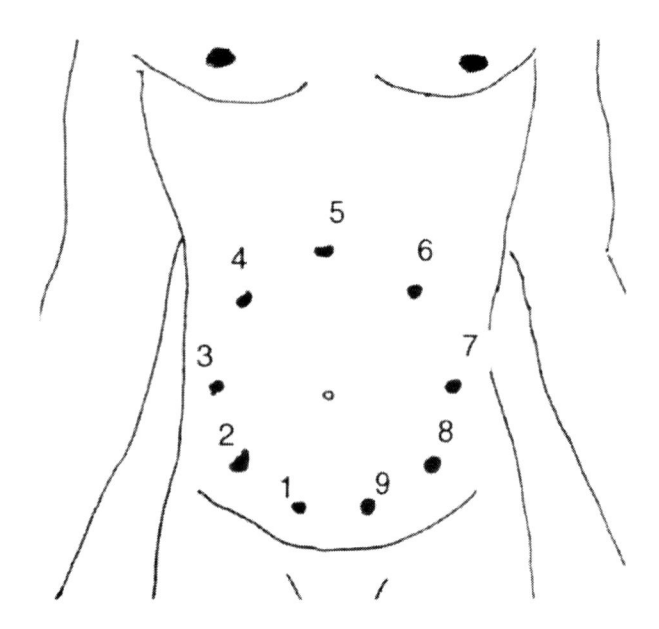

e. One hand or both hands can be used to do the points. If you use both hands, usually the right hand is at the bottom and the left hand is placed on top. The pressure is on the bottom hand while the top hand merely supports the bottom hand.

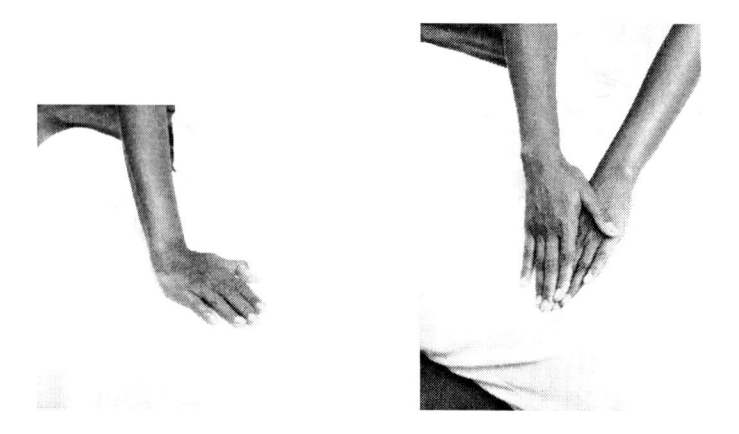

20 (e) Mixing the cauldron of the five elements

f. Kneeling on the right side of the receiver and facing point one, place one hand on point 1 and press down with the heel of the fingers, arm extended and elbow straight on Point 1, as the receiver inhales. Hold the position and the pressure of the heel of the hand in place.

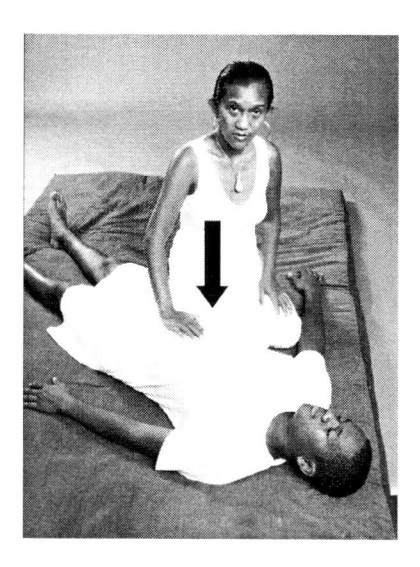

20 (f) Mixing the cauldron of the five elements

g. After the second time the receiver exhales, use the heel of your hand to push slowly, creating a wave toward the navel at the center of the circle. Pull back with the fingertips and slide all the way to the beginning of point 1. Feel the wave and work with the breath.

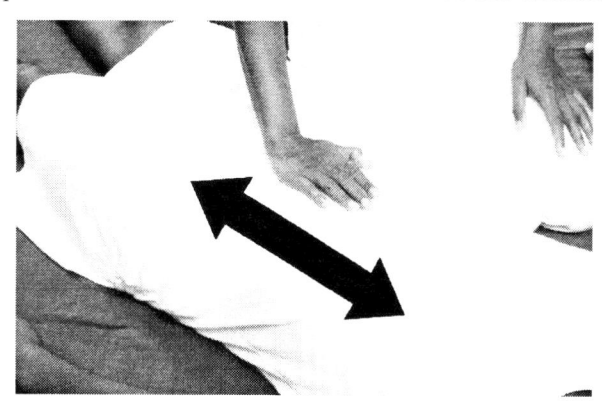

20 (g) Mixing the cauldron of the five elements

h. Proceed with **Point 2**, working in harmony with the breaths of the receiver. Coaching the receiver with the inhalation and exhalation rhythm helps to synchronize the movements. Press on exhalation.

If there's no consciousness of proper breathing on the receiver's part, the giver must breathe in proper rhythm to allow the waves to happen.

i. Keep changing your angle for comfort. Points 1-5 can be worked on the right side and the giver can switch to the left side for points 6-9.

The Healing Dance

It is recommended that Point 5 is worked on with the left hand as the giver remains on the right side.

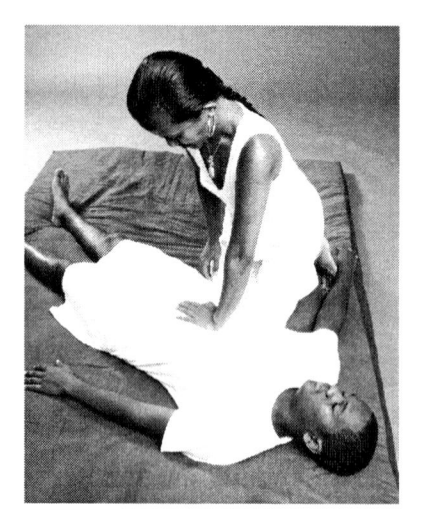

20 (i) Mixing the cauldron of the five elements

j. If the giver decides to stay on the right side to continue points 6-9, use the finger tips to press down on exhalation. Hold the pressure on inhalation, then on the next exhalation pull in towards navel. Push back with the heel and slide all the way to the beginning of the point with fingers extended. Again, feel the wave.

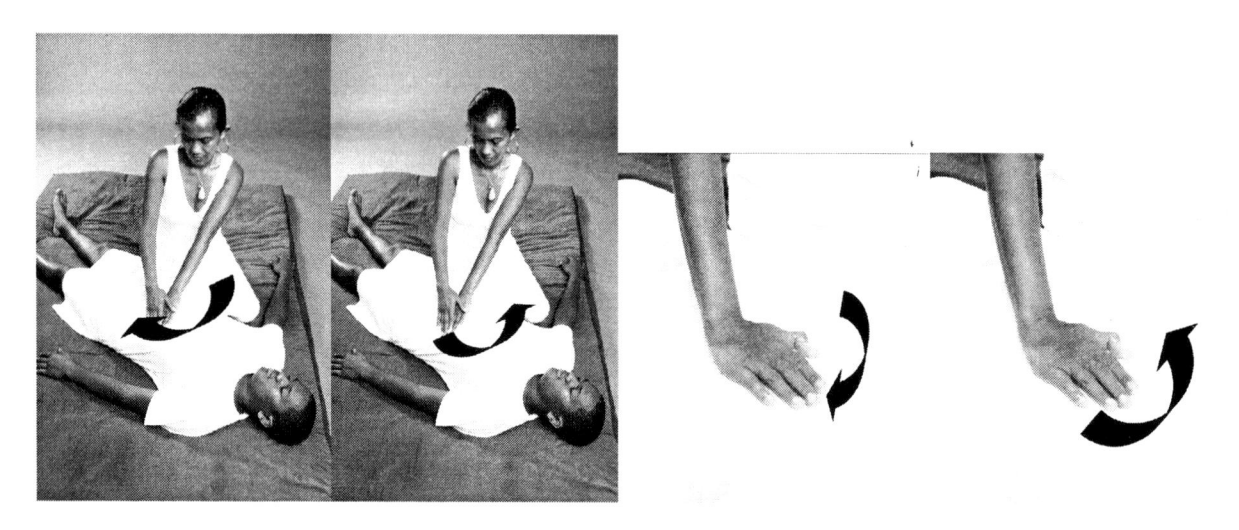

20 (j) Mixing the cauldron of the five elements

21. OPEN UP HEART AND LUNGS:
(SPIRAL DANCE OF THE FINGERS)

Fourth Chakra – Numbers 21-23

a. The giver may sit on the right or straddle for comfort. With the giver's three middle fingers, make three to five circles along the sternum from the lower end to center of the clavicle then down and back up again. As your finger completes the end of the third circle of each set, just let your fingers slide up to the next spot, do the three finger circles and slide up again, repeat the spiral cycle (up–down–up).

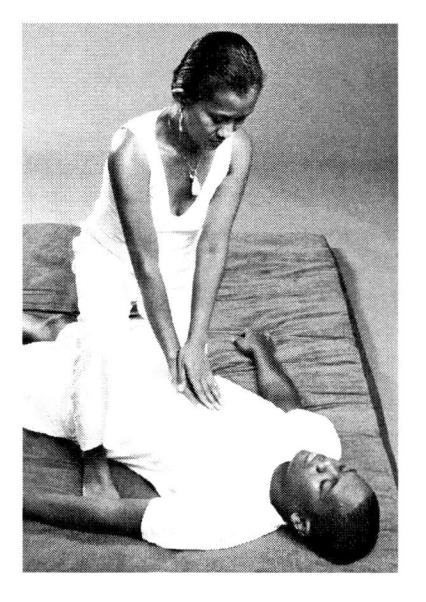

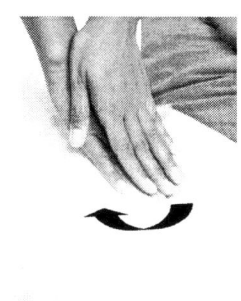

21 (a) Dancing snake

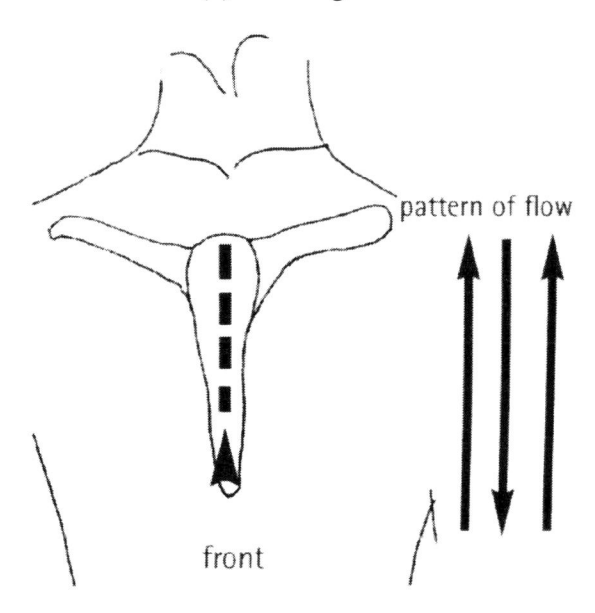

pattern of flow

front

b. Just below the center of the clavicle, the giver positions both hands side by side to continue three sets of finger circles with clockwise circles of the right hand and counterclockwise circles with the left hand. Gradually move from the center to mid-clavicle to outer clavicle back to mid-clavicle and to the center (repeat x2.5 cycles and on the outer clavicle).

The Healing Dance 61

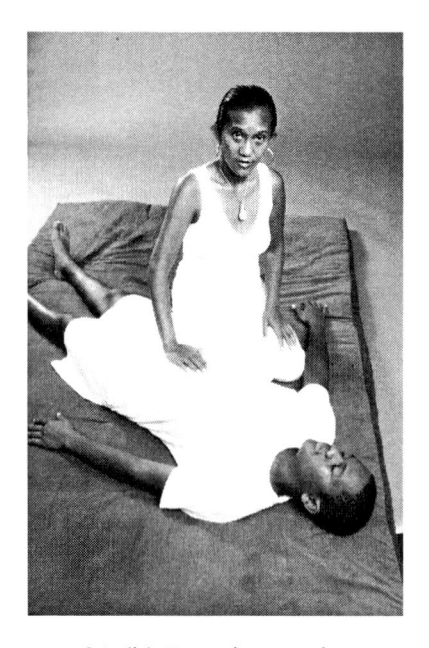

21 (b) Dancing snake

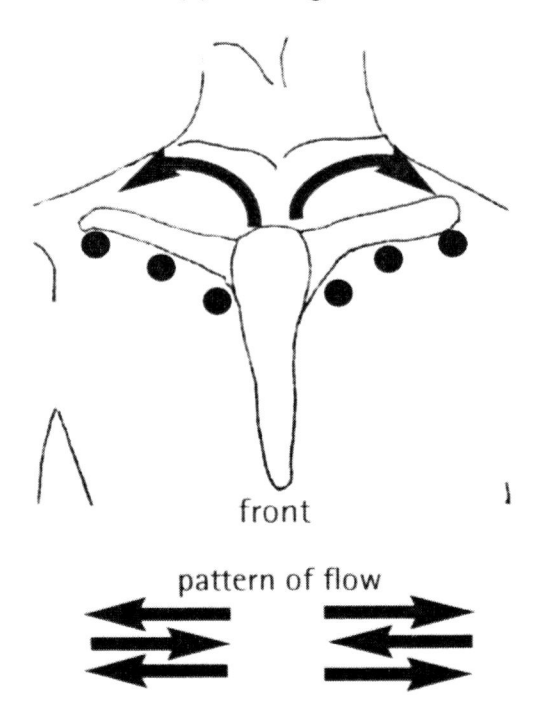

front

pattern of flow

22. PRESS, HOOK AND PULL SHOULDERS:

a. The giver places the heel of each hand on the muscular part below the outer clavicle. The giver keeps elbows straight, rocks toward the floor, and rocks back and pulls with the fingers to hook at the back of the shoulder opposite the heel of the palm. The shoulders get lifted upward. Follow with three finger circles after lift.

Continue with the movement toward the neck. (From the outer to the middle shoulder, to the neck and back to the middle shoulder and outer shoulder).

Do three finger circles each lift.

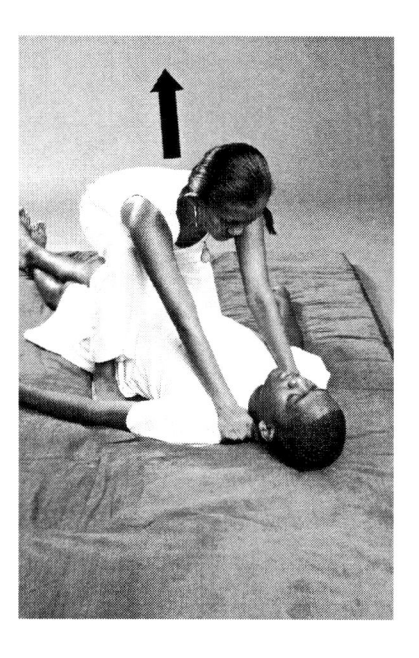

22 (a) Eagle catches prey

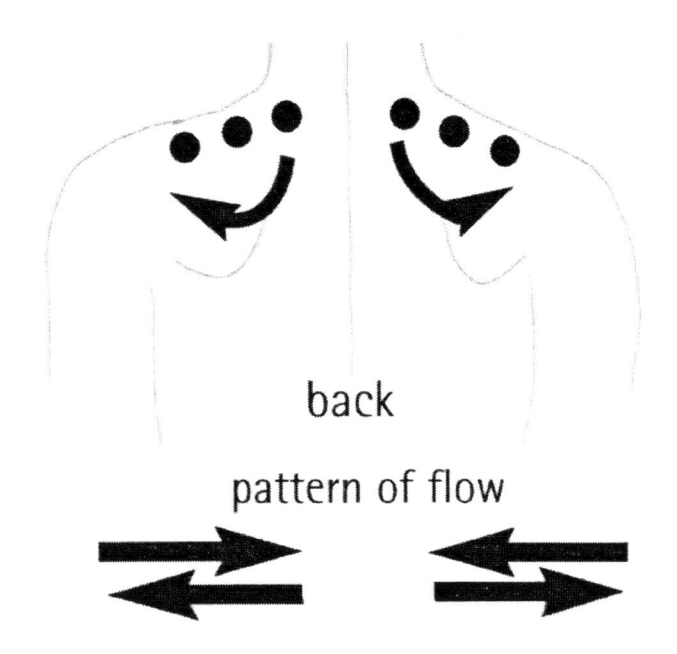

back

pattern of flow

b. Alternate palm-press arms from upper arm down to the hands. Stretch simultaneously both hands with palms up.

The Healing Dance 63

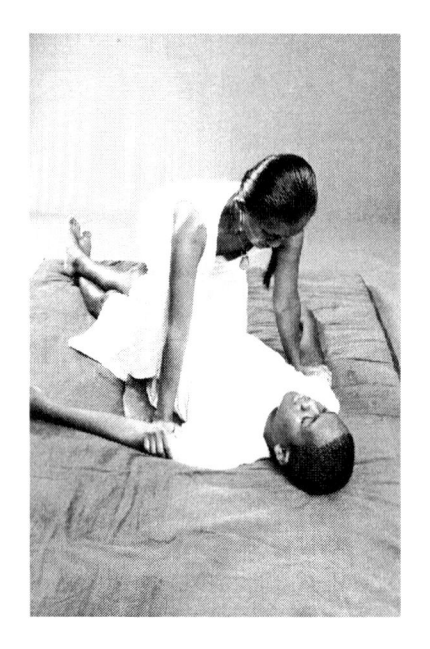

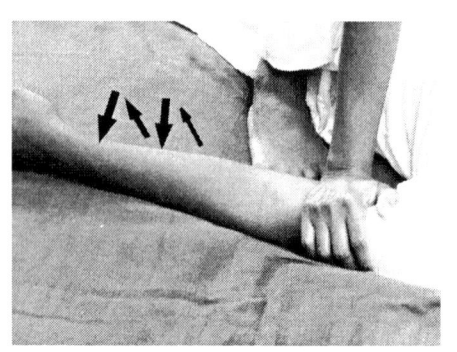

22 (b) Clearing the barrier

23. HEAD, NECK AND FACE-FRONT POSITION

Fifth Chakra

a. The giver kneels and alternately palm presses the shoulder in a rocking motion.

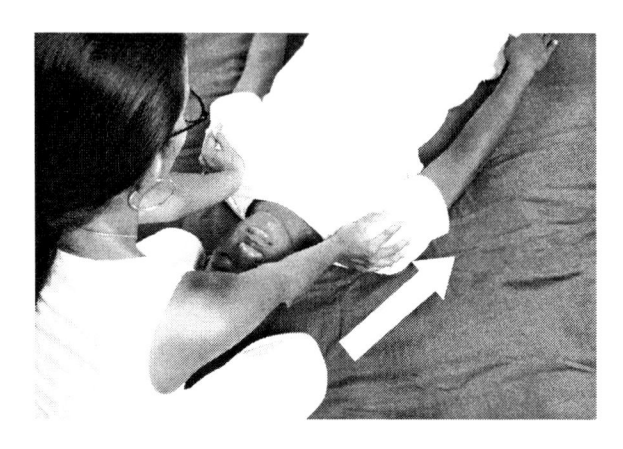

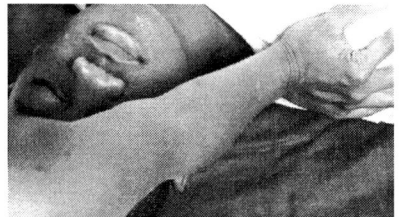

23 (a) Unlock Lotus

b. CRADLE THE NECK:

Cradle the neck with one hand while the other hand palm-presses from neck to mid-shoulder to outer shoulder and back again (soft-hard-soft).

The hand that cradles the neck can provide traction for a greater stretch. Do this three times on each side.

c. CHIN UP—CHIN DOWN

Hook one or two fingers from each hand under the neck along the side of transverse processes in the cervical vertebrae alongside the neck. Rock forward, lift up on the neck and pull towards you sliding the fingers over the head gently as you sit upright and reposition your fingers/hands all the way up to the occipital ridge. Repeat the process as you adjust the position of your fingers moving towards the occipital ridge. The chin and the neck flex and extend gracefully.

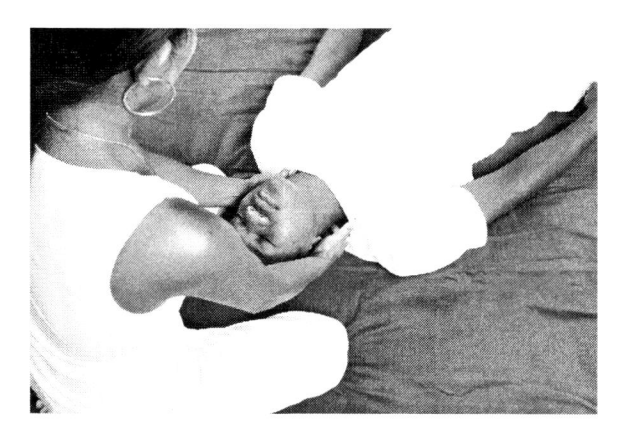

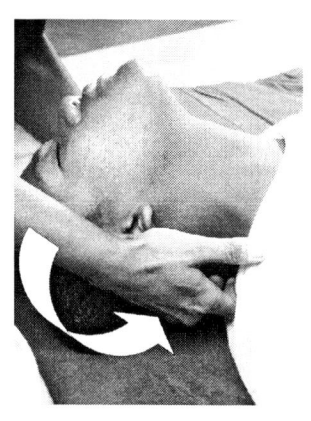

23 (c) Gather dreams

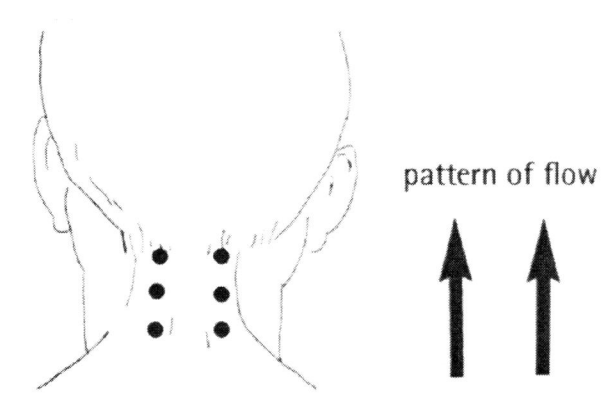

pattern of flow

d. At the occipital ridge, with both hands together, rock forward gently as you lift and rock back and pull from the center to the outer edge and back.

The Healing Dance 65

Fifth, Sixth and Seventh Chakras

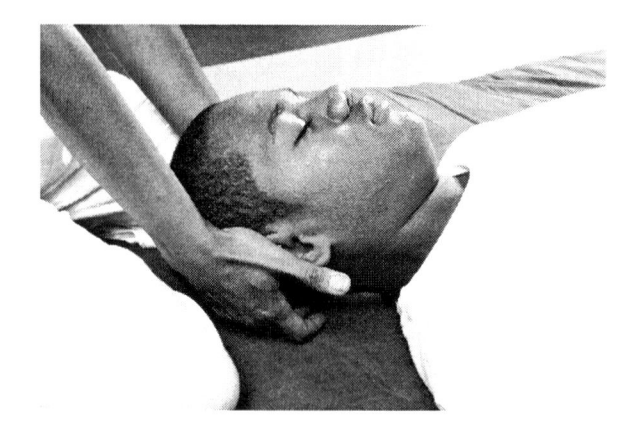

23 (d) Gather dreams

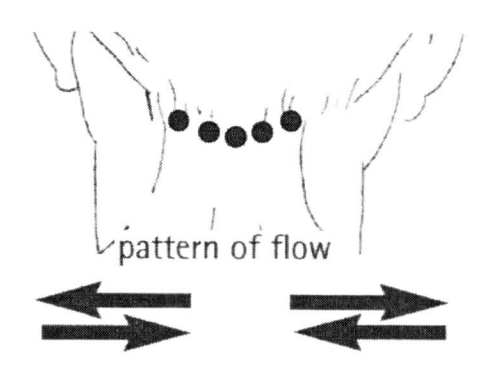

e. With one hand cradling the head, turn the head to one side and perform finger circles along the side of the neck from outer to the middle to the center and back to the middle and outer areas. Three finger circles on each point will be sufficient.

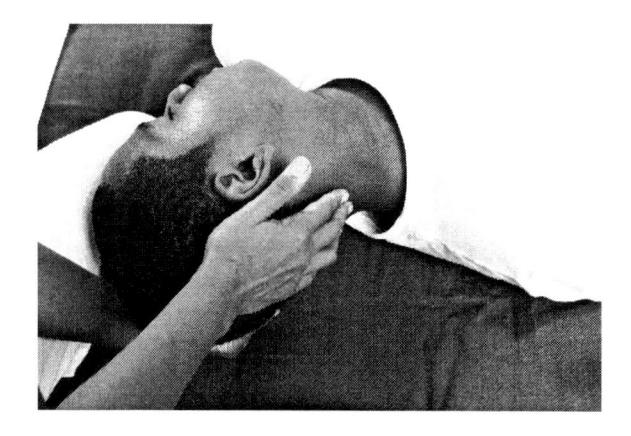

23 (e) Gather dreams

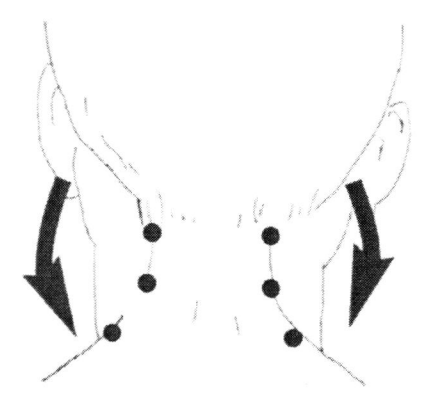

f. From the occipital ridge, finger-walk up the centerline of the crown of the head and thumb-walk the centerline all the way to the top of the hairline. At the hairline, walk down thumb-over-thumb to the crown and thumb-on-thumb back to hairline.

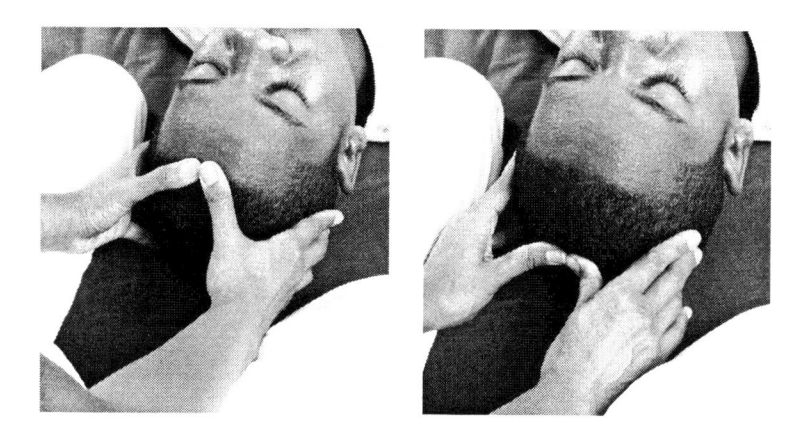

23 (f) Gather dreams

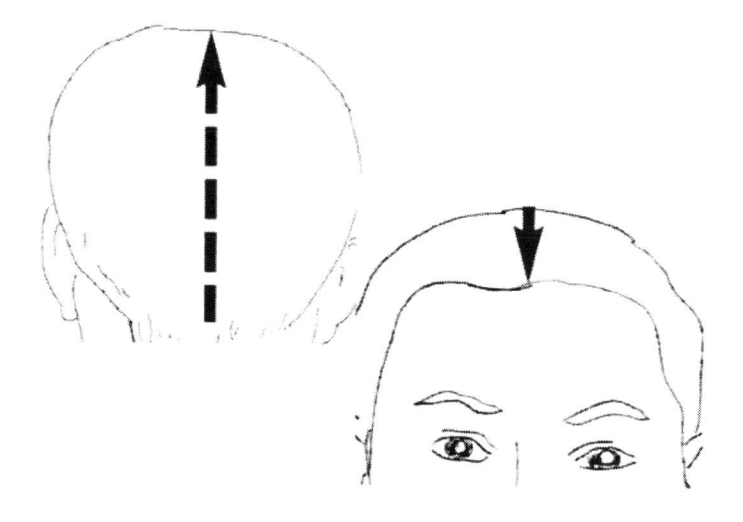

g. Dry-shampoo the scalp with fingertip circles around the entire scalp.

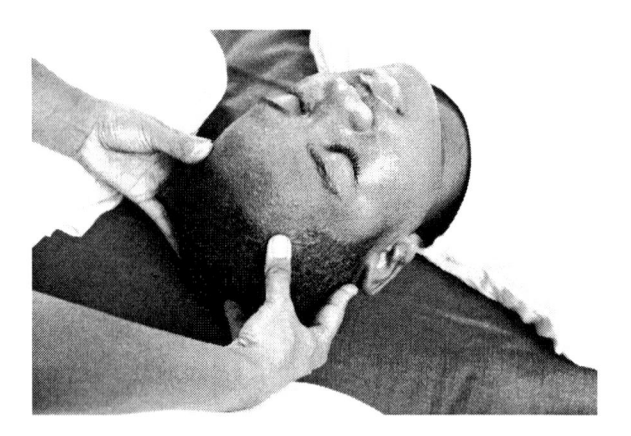

23 (g) Gather dreams

h. Make small thumb circles along the lines of the forehead starting from the center and sliding the thumbs to the temples, closing the lines with thumb circles.

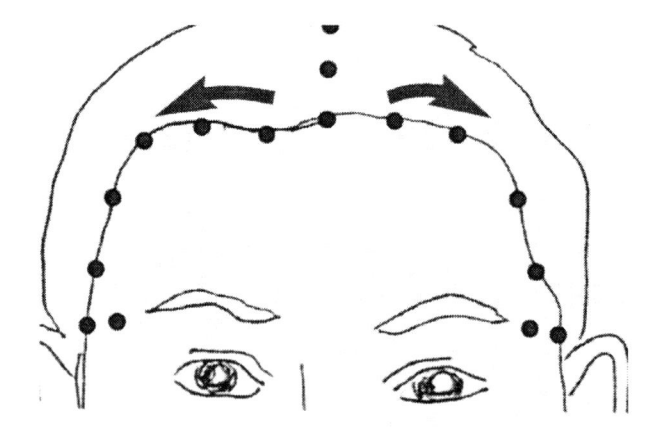

i. Repeat the process moving down from the hairline closer to the eyebrows.

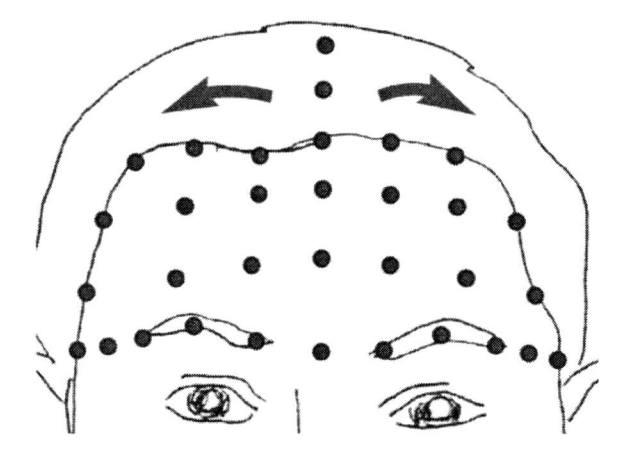

j. Make fingertip circles around the eyes. Close with circles on the temples.

68 *Grace Sunga Asagra*

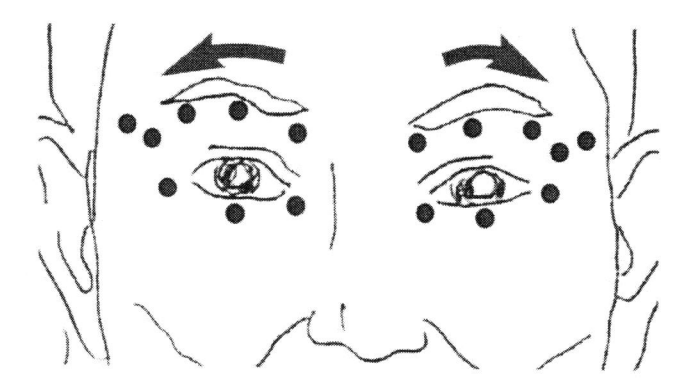

k. Continue the process on the cheekbones and toward the bottom of the jawbone. Use a gentle pinching and lifting movement all the way to the ear-lobes. Every line ends at the temple with circles except for the jaw pinch and pull move.

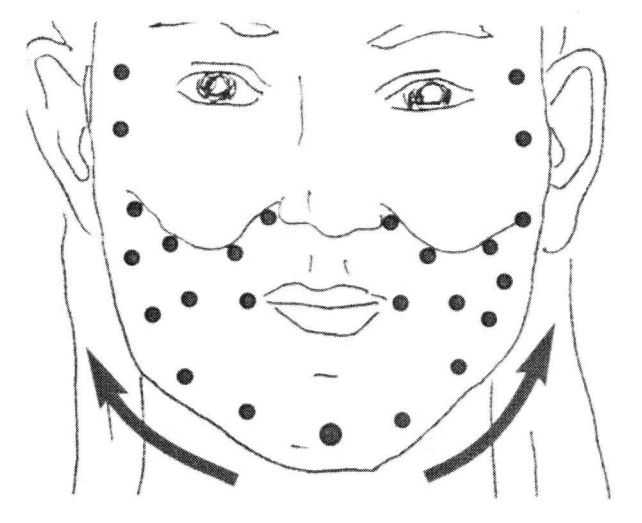

l. Pull downward gently on the earlobes and massage the ears. Cup the hands over the ears and hold for a minute, then do finger circles around the borders of the ears.

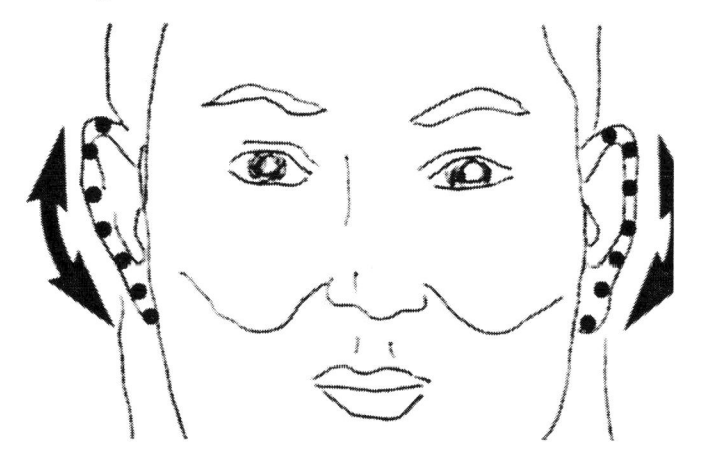

m. Turn the head from side to side and stretch the neck.

The Healing Dance 69

n. Twist the head from side to side and stretch the neck.

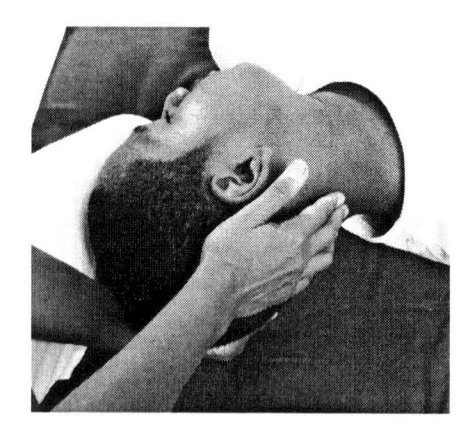

23 (n) Gather dreams

24. CLOSING THE LOOP

First to Fifth Chakras

a. The receiver turns over on the back. The giver repeats alternate palm-presses up and down the legs.

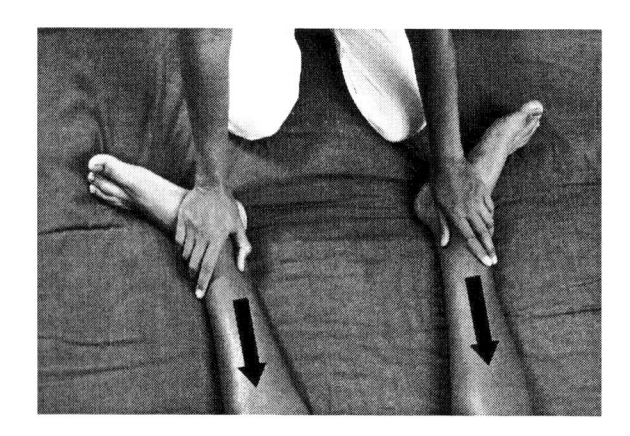

24 (a) Stimulate yin and yang

b. Place the receiver's extended legs on your side, adjacent to the giver's hips. Grab each other's forearms, pull and lean back. Do this 3 times.

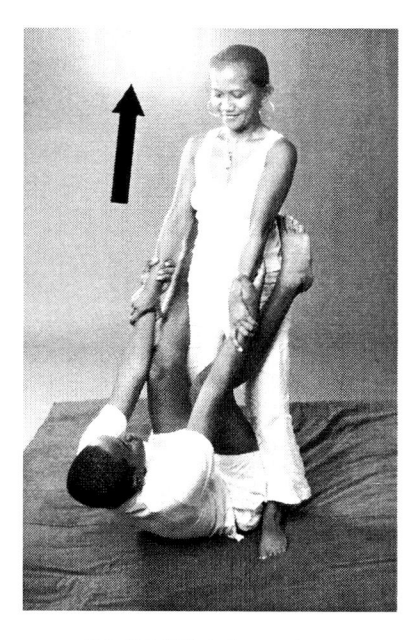

24 (b) Weigh anchor

Yoga Nindra
Preliminary to foot prayer pose.

c. The receiver crosses his legs in front and below the giver's knees as the receiver's feet are positioned close to receiver's buttocks. Both grab each other's hands and giver pulls upward three times. On the third time, the giver takes small steps backward and pulls the receiver into a sitting position.

Urdhva Padmasana in Sirsasana

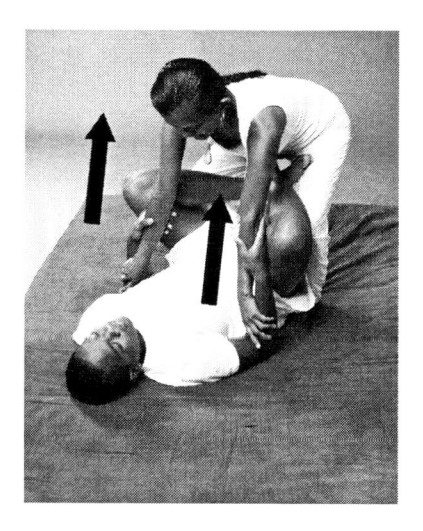

24 (c) Cracking open walnut

The Healing Dance 71

II. SIDE POSITION:

First, Second and Third Chakras

1. Side position of the male receiver begins on the right side with the right leg straight (bottom leg) and the left leg bent (top leg). Do the opposite for a female receiver. She lies on her left side, left leg (bottom leg straight) and right leg (top leg) bent. Adjust the support on the neck for comfort. Provide a pillow for the receiver to cuddle and to keep him from rolling onto his abdomen.

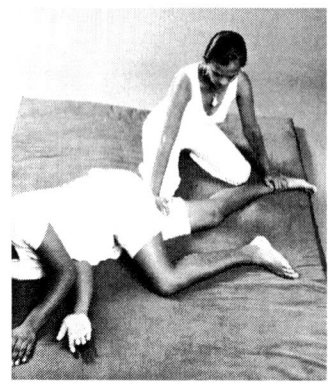

1. Moving mountain

2. The giver kneels in front of the legs, rocks side to side and alternately palm-presses from ankles to the hips and back down.

3. MOVING MOUNTAINS

a. The giver shifts position on the receiver's back. The giver stretches the bottom leg, which is the straight leg, with one hand on the thigh and the other hand on the ankle. The giver then rocks and alternately palm-presses in toward the knees, then out to the thigh and ankle, then in toward the knees.

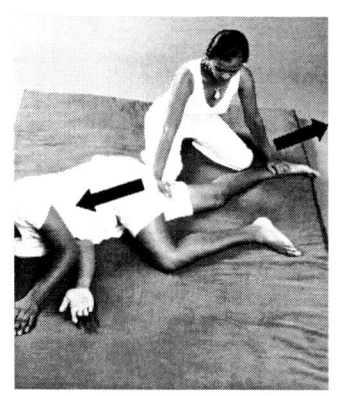

3. Moving mountain

pattern of flow

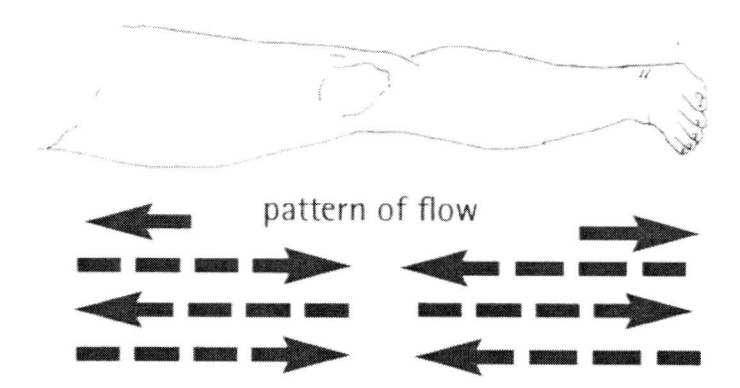

b. With both hands, alternate palm-press from the knee to the ankle and alternate palm-press up to the thigh and down to the ankle, with a stretch of the ankle at the end.

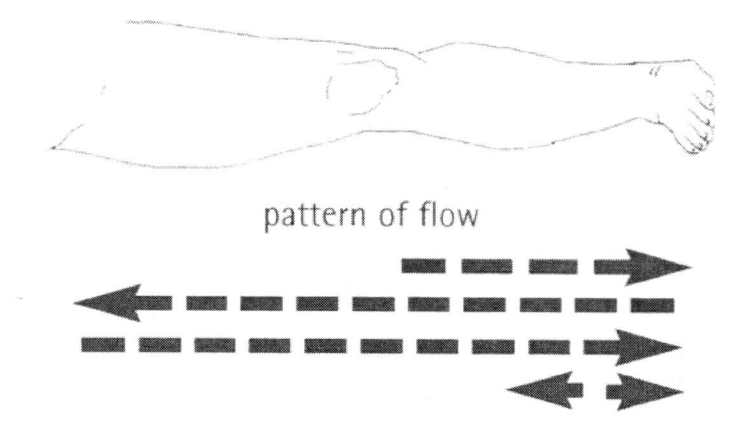

pattern of flow

4. While in a half-kneeling position, the giver's outer leg is raised between the receiver's legs while the giver's other leg is kneeling at the back of the receiver's straight leg. The giver stretches the bent top leg in three parts.

a. Stretch from **hip** to ankle.

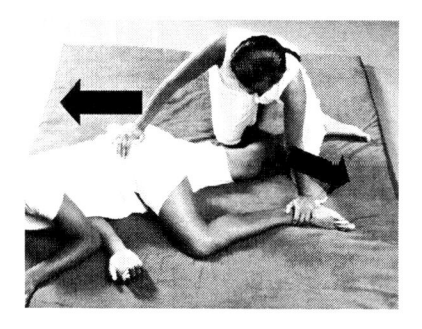

b. Stretch from **knee** to ankle.

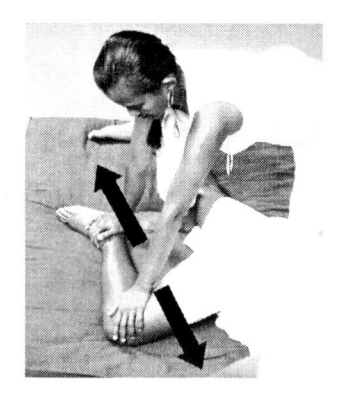

c. Stretch from hip to knee.

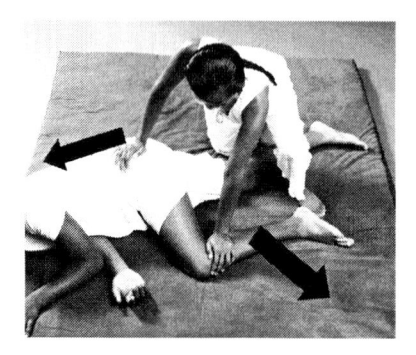

5. Back to rocking and alternate palm-presses with one hand starting from the hip and the other, starting from the ankle to the knee, then out to the hip and ankle, then back to the knee.

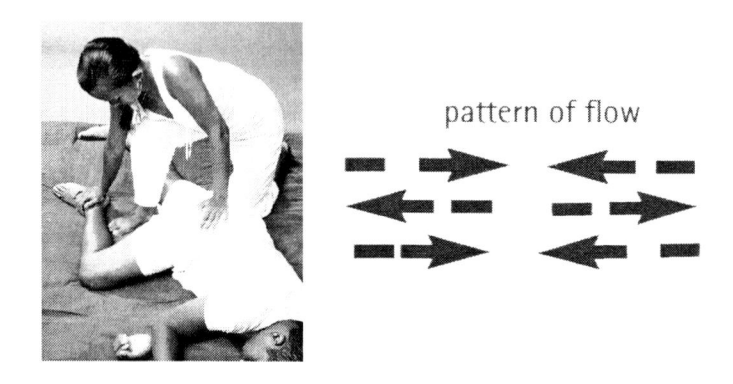

pattern of flow

5. Moving mountains

74 *Grace Sunga Asagra*

6. Both hands alternate palm-presses down to the foot and back up to the hip and down to foot with a stretch of the ankle at the end.

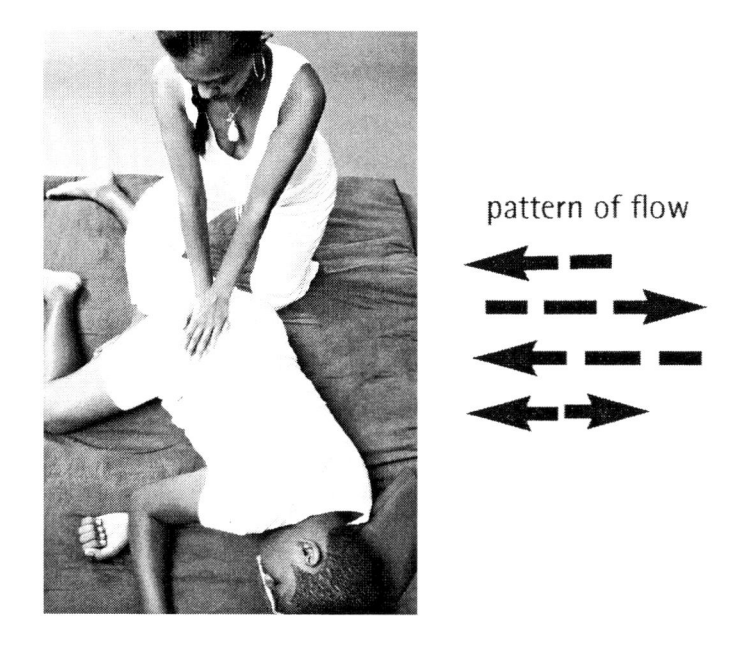

pattern of flow

6. Moving mountains

7. HIP POINTS

a. Alternate palm-presses from the ankles up to the hips.

b. Big palm circle on the trochanter.

c. Palm-press the three points (triangle points) with either the heel of your hand or fingertips finding the three points finger press for five seconds, then finger-circle each point, then palm-circle the area. You can feel the indentations once you press the points. Be gentle because these points are tender for most people.

The Healing Dance

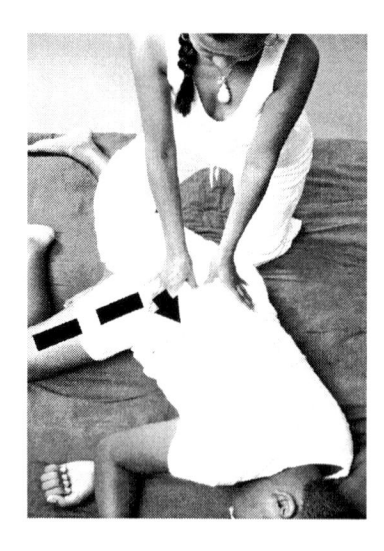

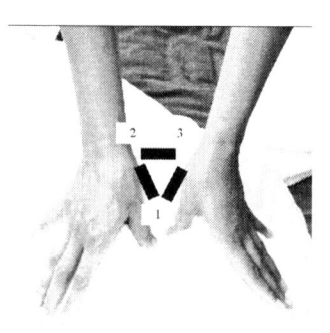

7 (c) Moving mountains

8. SPINE WORK

Rock side-to-side and alternate palm-press on the outer border of the spine from the waist up and down.

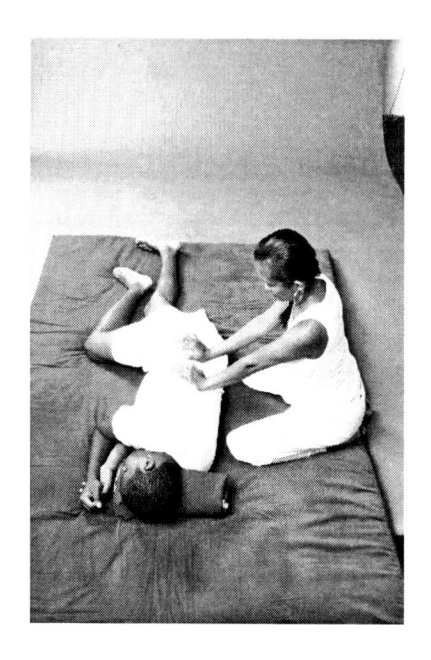

8. Cultivating the land

9. SHOULDER WORK

Fourth and Fifth Chakras

a. With giver's hand closest to the receiver's top shoulder, reach the receiver's arm. Hold with one hand and palm circle around the scapula.

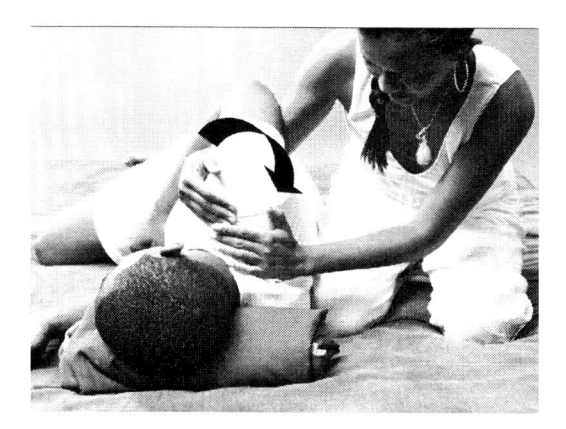

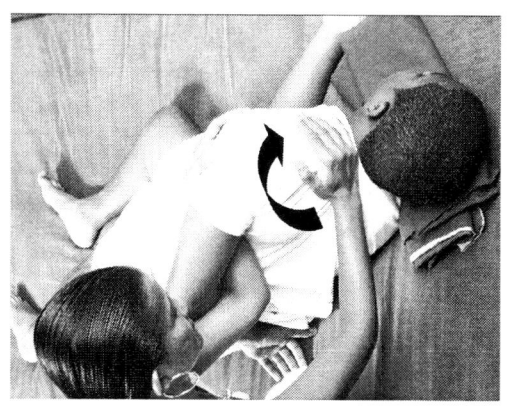

9 (a) Cultivating the land

b. Thumb circle the scapula while the other hand pushes the shoulder down.

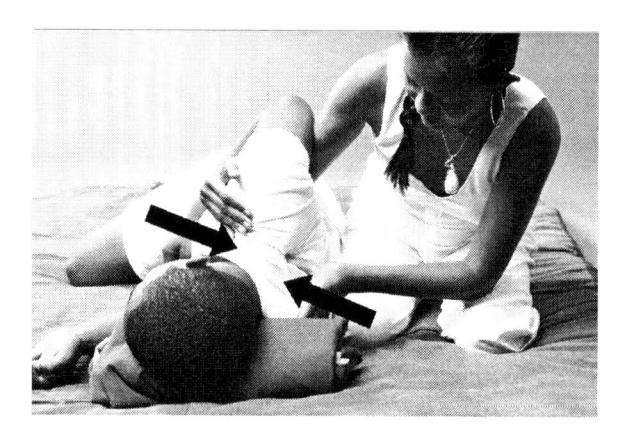

9 (b) Cultivating the land

c. Repeat palm circles around the shoulder area.

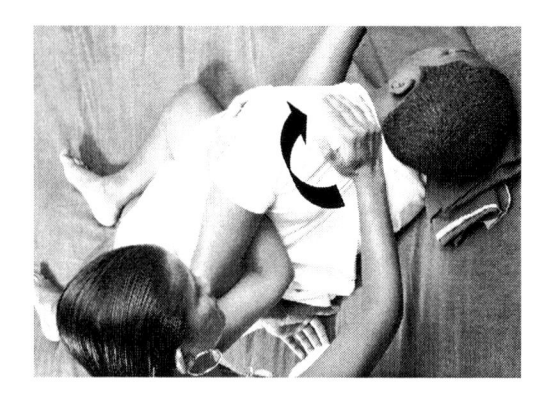

9 (c) Cultivating the land

d. While in a half-kneeling position (right knee) and with your outer left hand hold and raise the right hand of the receiver above and over the head while your other hand holds the right axilla (armpit area) and the right lateral side of the receiver's chest. Make three good stretches (First position is the palm of the hand on the axilla, second position is just a palm down from the axilla, and the third is two palms below the axilla).

Repeat on the other side of the receiver with giver on a half-kneeling position (left knee), outer right hand hold and raise the left hand of the receiver above and over the head.

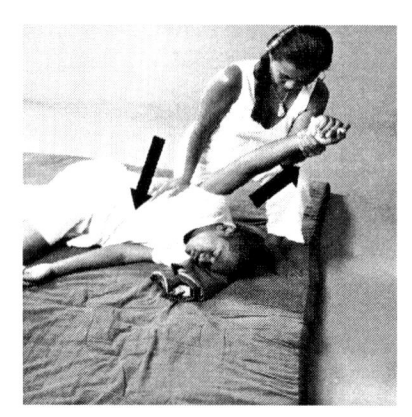

9 (d) Cultivating the land

III. PRONE POSITION

"I got your back"

1. SOLE-TO-SOLE

a. "Soul-to-Soul" with sole-to-sole movement with the receiver's back facing away from the receiver. The receiver alternately steps and rocks from one sole to the other. Do not walk on the heels.

Grace Sunga Asagra

Resting cobra pose.

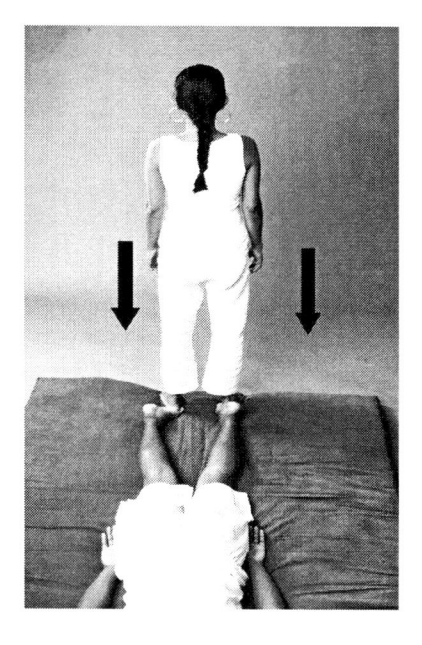

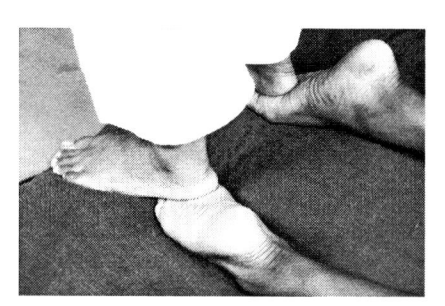

1 (a) Stretching the roots

2. SOLE-TO-SOLE

a. Face the receiver and walk on the arch and ball, using the balls of the receiver's feet.

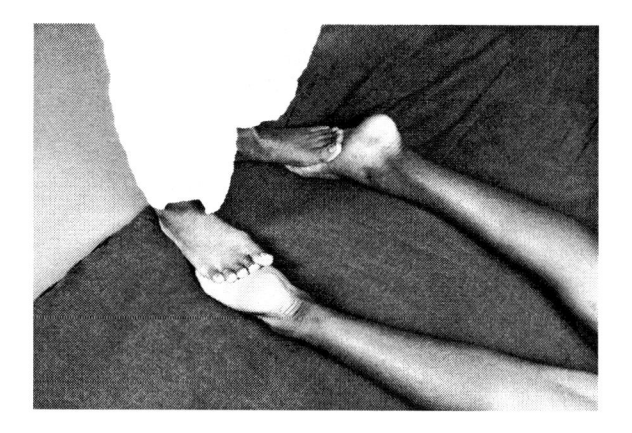

2 (a) Stretching the roots

SPLITTING BAMBOO

b. The giver kneels on the receiver's sole and rocks with the knees.

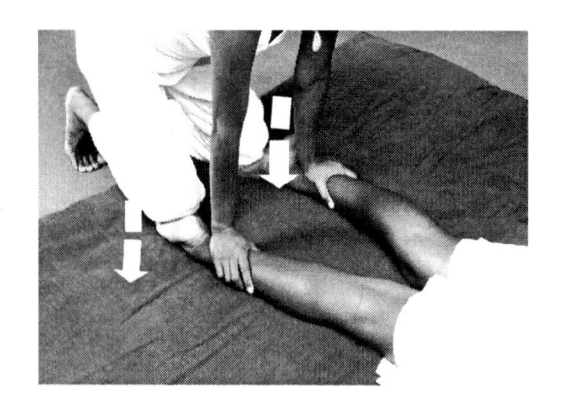

2 (b) Splitting bamboo

3. CROSSING A BAMBOO BRIDGE

a. The giver kneels on the ground and rocks side to side with fists on the receiver's sole. The giver's knees are used to maintain balance in coordination with the fists.

4. ELEPHANT WALKING

First and Second Chakras
a. The giver kneels facing the receiver's back and rocks and alternate palm-presses from the ankles up the legs to the gluteal fold, then back to the ankles.

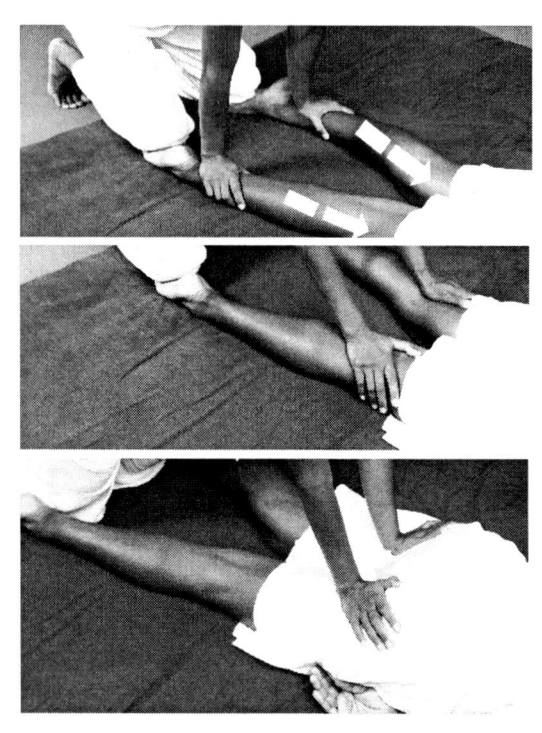

4 (a) Splitting Bamboo

b. Rock and alternate thumb-press up and down the centerline of the calf and thigh. Be gentle on the calf because of its increased sensitivity for most individuals.

c. Repeat rocking from side to side with alternate palm-press from the ankle to the gluteal fold.

Yoga Nindra

Hold the pressure on the pulse spot on gluteal fold; raise your body as you hold the pressure for 30-60 seconds.

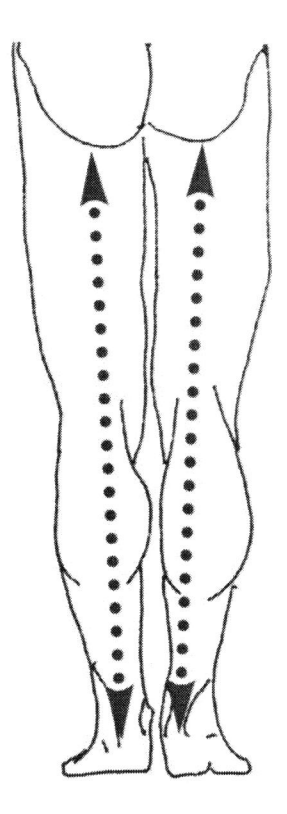

5. ROCK THE BOAT

First, Second and Third Chakras

a. While in a kneeling position, hold the receiver's feet. Bend the legs and, starting from ankles, rock and press your feet to gluteal three times, moving the hands from the ankles to the toes and down the ankles. (Soft pressure-on ankles, medium pressure halfway, and hard pressure on the toes, then back to medium-halfway, then to soft on ankles).

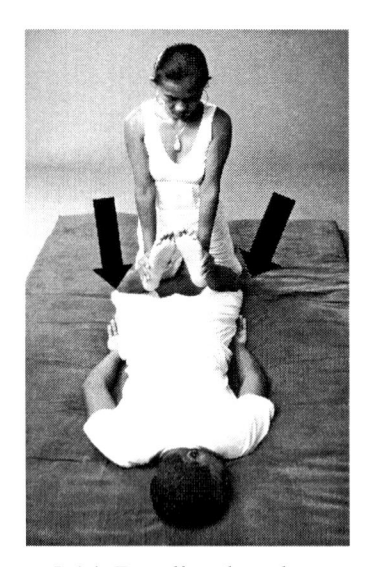

5 (a) Bending bamboo

b. Place a foot on top of each of the receiver's feet. Rock and press the ankles toward the gluteus maximus, moving the hands up to toes with each press and down to the ankles. Reverse crossing of feet and repeat.

Preliminary to a bow pose.

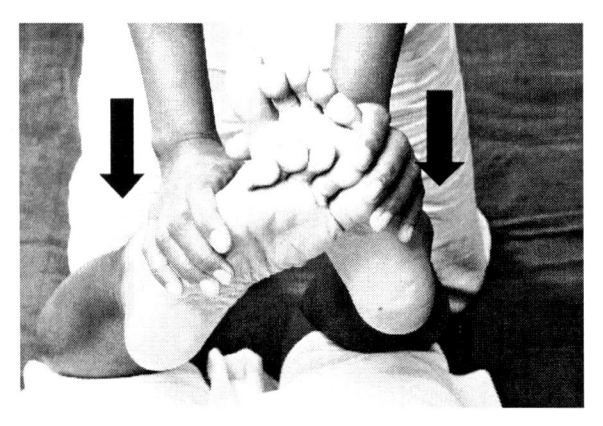

5 (b) Twisting the roots

6. UPPER BACK-Pumping the legs

First to Sixth Chakras

a. With the receiver's legs bent and feet raised, the giver sits on the receiver's feet and palm press together the spinous processes- the two bony protrusions on the posterior side of each vertebrae along the spine - from waist up, then alternate palm-presses back to the waist. The giver's hands are pointing upward. When the giver sits on the receiver soles, the giver must position her own feet close to the axilla.

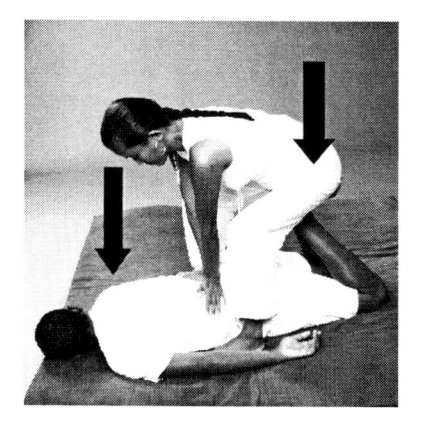

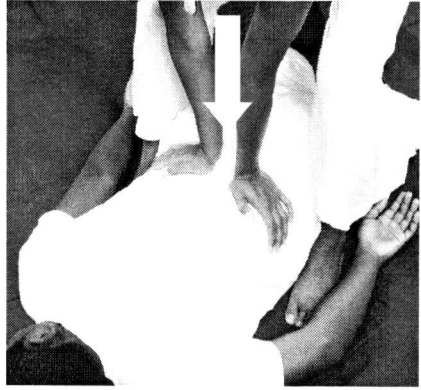

6 (a) Rocking the gate

b. Thumb-press together along the spine from waist up and alternate thumb-press down.

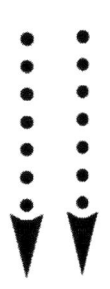

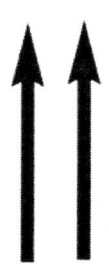

c. At the waist, starting along the spine, thumb-press together the iliac crest – long curved upper border of the ilium which is the uppermost and largest bone on the pelvis. Do this three times, moving out and then back in. Thumb circle at the end of each thumb-press.

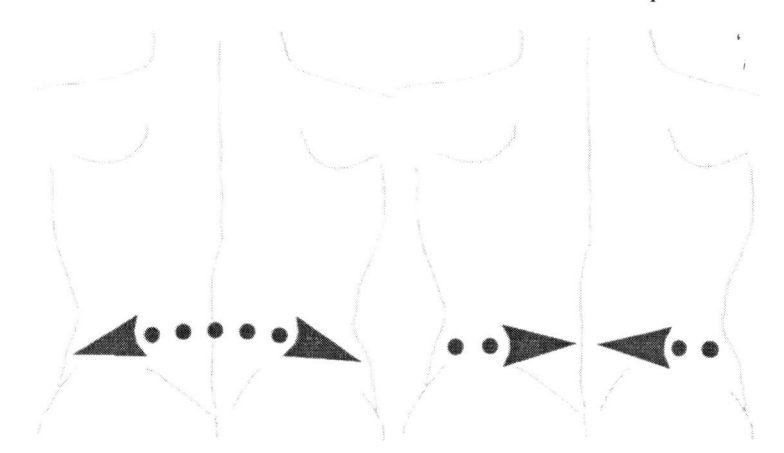

d. Repeat palm-press together up the shoulder along the spine and alternate palm-press back to the waist.

The Healing Dance 83

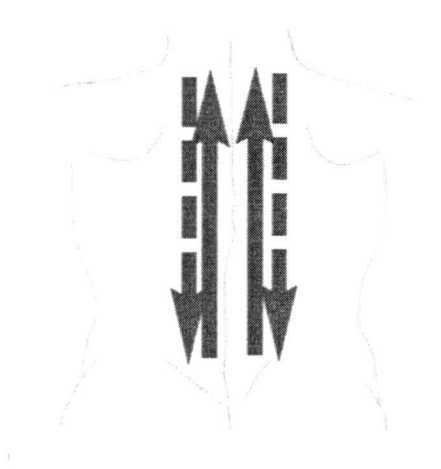

7. CLOSING THE LOOP

First to Fifth Chakras

a. The receiver turns over on the back; the giver repeats alternate palm-press up and down the legs.

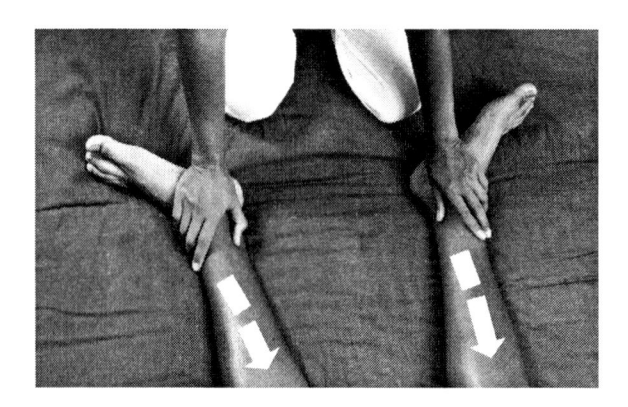

7 (a) Stimulate yin and yang

b. Place the receiver's extended legs on your sides adjacent to your hips. Grab each other's forearms, pull and lean back. Do this three times.

Yoga Nindra
Preliminary to foot prayer pose.

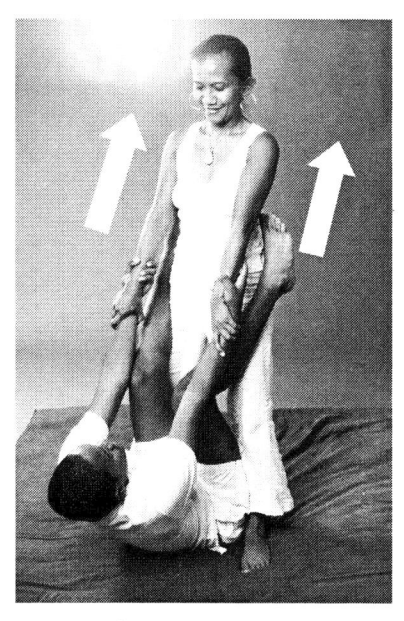

7 (b) Weigh anchor

c. Cross the receiver legs in front and below your knees as the receiver's feet are positioned close to receiver's buttocks. Grab each other's hands and pull upwards three times. On the third time, the giver takes small steps backward and pulls the receiver into a sitting position.

Urdhva Padmasana in Sirsasana

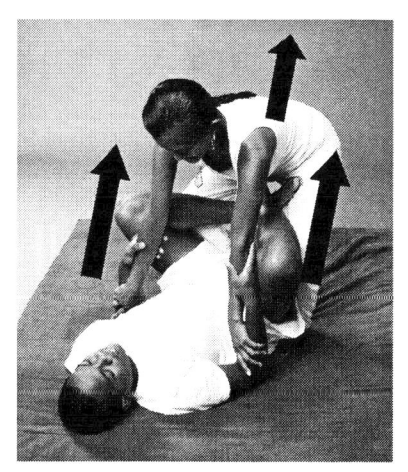

7 (c) Cracking open walnut

The Healing Dance 85

IV. Sitting

First, Fifth and Seventh Chakras

1. SITTING MONKEY
a. The giver stands behind the receiver and supports the receiver's back gently with the knees. The giver places her hands with fingers pointing down the back at the junction of the neck and shoulders. Palm-press together three times from the neck out to the shoulders and then back to the neck.

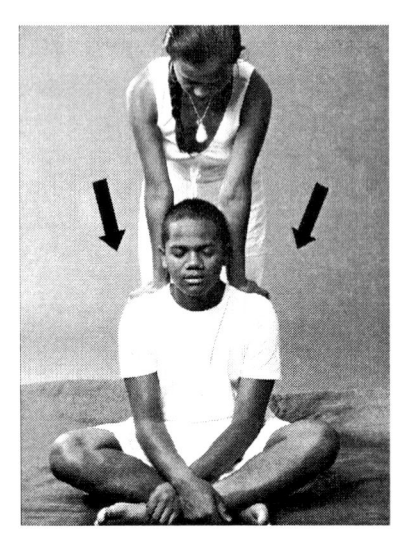

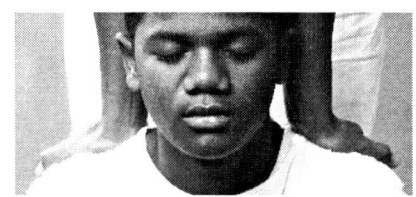

1 (a) Lotus pose

2. Reposition the hands with fingers pointing towards the chest, except for the thumbs. Palm press together three times from the neck out to the shoulder.

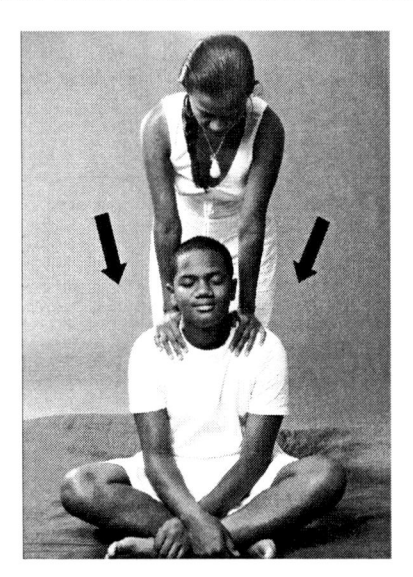

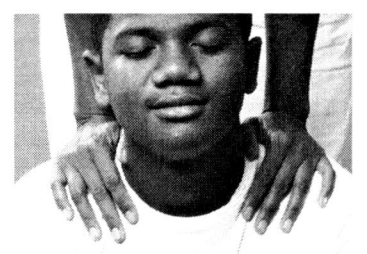

2. Lotus pose

86 *Grace Sunga Asagra*

3. Thumb-press together the points along the shoulder from the neck to the outer border. Shift thumbs down slightly lower on the trapezius and thumb-press back to the neck. Hold each point for five seconds. Release with a thumb circle in each thumb-press.

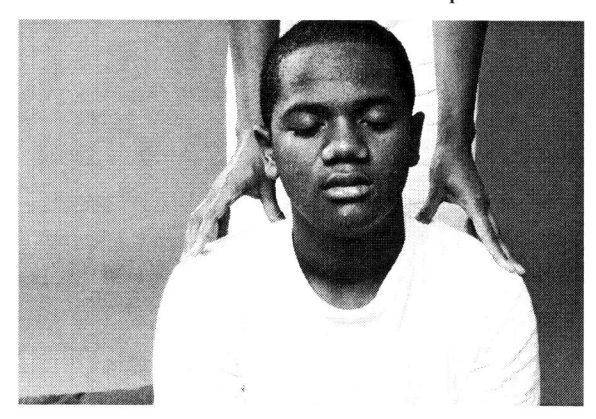

3. Lotus pose

4. As the giver kneels behind the receiver's back, place both thumbs on the hollow on the sides of the neck along the spine. The receiver drops his elbows slightly for more pressure. Work up and down the neck two times.

5. Interlace fingers. Work the same area using the heels of the palms to squeeze and lift along the neck. Close by using thumb and fingers to squeeze and knead the area.

All Chakras

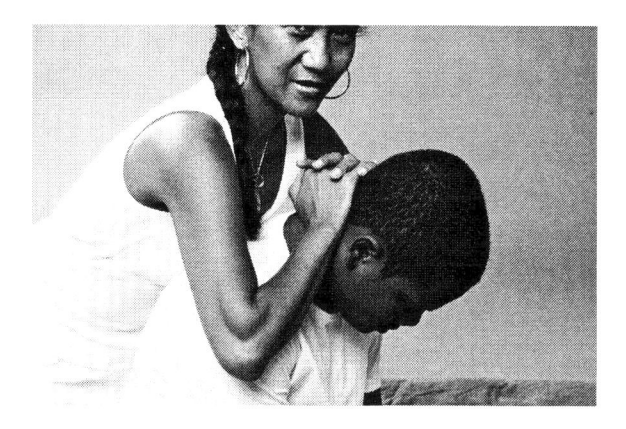

5. Lotus pose

6. Chop out shoulder, and along the spine going down to the waist and back up. Repeat on the other side. Do not chop on the kidneys and bones. Palm circle the entire back. Brush three to five times down to the back and out to the side.

The Healing Dance 87

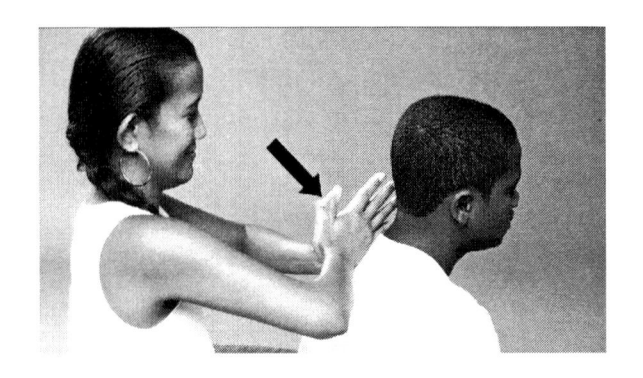

6. Lotus pose

7. Subtle Bodies

Assist the receiver to sit up in a lotus position when possible. Kneel behind the receiver's back. WITHOUT TOUCHING THE RECEIVER'S PHYSICAL BODY do the following as a closure:

(Points A)
a. Move your hands horizontally, sweeping the energy from the upper-middle to the lateral side of the back of the receiver.

(Points B)
b. Second sweep is on the energy on the mid-back section from the middle to the lateral side of the back of the receiver.

(Points C)
c. Third sweep is on the lower back from the lower middle to the lateral side of the back of the receiver.

(Points D)
d. Fourth sweep is from the back of the shoulder to the waist of the receiver's back.

(Points E)
e. Fifth sweep. The hands move up in an E position to the crown chakra.

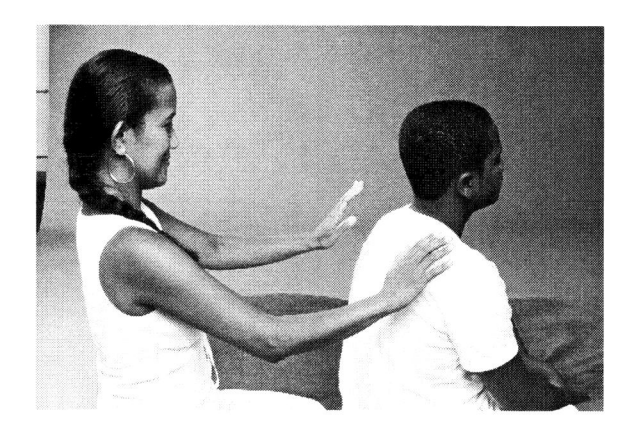

7. Lotus pose

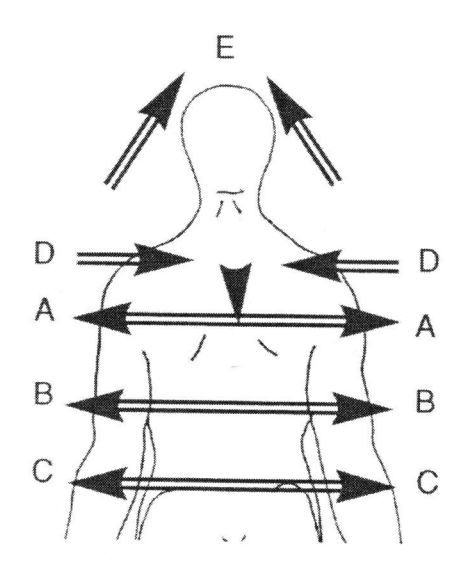

8. Rest one **hand on** the receiver's back opposite the heart and the other hand on the giver's heart.

The Healing Dance 89

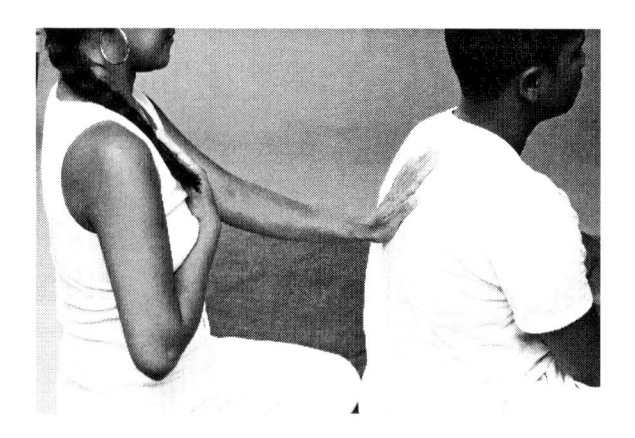

8. Heart to heart

9. Face the receiver, place hands on a prayer position, smile and say, Sawadee to a male receiver and Sawadee ka to a female receiver. It is a warm greeting in Thai. You can also choose another greeting or prayer at the end.

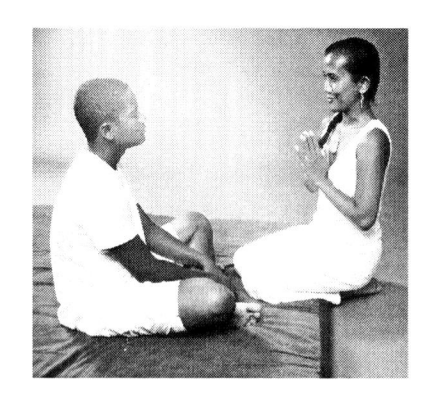

9. Lotus pose

Thank You

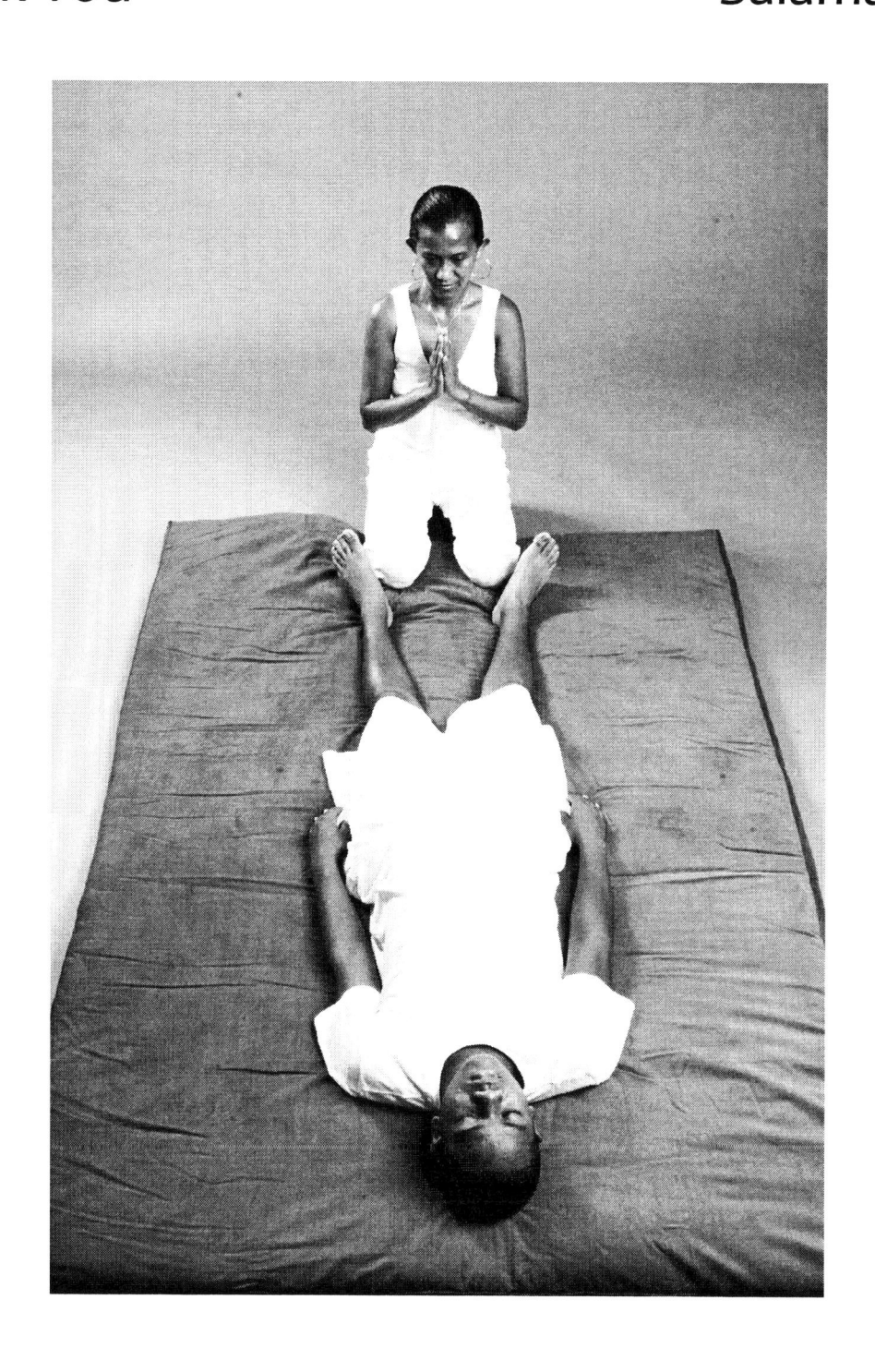

Salamat Po

The Healing Dance

Forces in Nature   Diwata

    In cultural ways of knowing, there are certain things that are difficult to put into words to explain to someone who has no experience with that culture. In my journey, information came to me from various cultural ways of knowing that have a direct connection with Filipino diwata, so I have included this introduction to diwata, for those who are unfamiliar with the concept.

    In the Philippine indigenous tradition, diwata are forces or energy in nature that serve as guides (deities or angels). The number and names of many diwata vary from region to region. It is believed that there is a force in everything. These forces not only exist in the external environment that we live in, but they are also manifested in our bodies, our internal environment. The teaching "as above, so below" (on earth as it is in heaven) brings wisdom to the mystery or magic of life not as separate, disconnected or fragmented, but belonging, connected or whole. Not as an outside observer, but as a participant observer and a co-creator in harmony with forces in nature.

    This section focuses on understanding the relationship of diwata with diseases that originates in the lower diwata at the base of the spine. It is an energy point that creates physiological reaction balanced by the parasympathetic and sympathetic nervous system and the adrenal gland affecting vital signs like blood pressure, blood sugar and processes like suppression of the immune system or over-activation of the immune system.

    Most diseases stem from our ability or inability to adapt. When stress, insecurity, fear, danger or an emergency occur we normally express ourselves through fight or flight (avoidance) response. This response is controlled by the autonomic nervous system and influences the internal organs (viscera) such as heart, stomach, intestine, uterus, and prostate glands. If this response occurs over a length of time, consciously or unconsciously, depending on the person or situation, it can create some serious problems affecting health and wellness.

    Fight and flight, or "survival of the fittest," as it is often expressed, are dual forces that habitually manifest in our lives. This is where a hilot would teach or recommend movements or techniques found in martial arts, yoga, tai-chi, qi-gong, drawing, cultural dance or meditation to help create effective ways of transformation that respond after a healing session. They would work to bring the person to the "rest and digest" response in the autonomic nervous system, where he or she could then connect to the parasympathetic nervous system where healing takes place.

These forces are neither good nor bad. They are forces that can help us move toward balance, growth, health and wellbeing. However, chronic habitual pattern of these forces lead to energies being stuck and blocked. Growth is stunted and signs and symptoms manifest, such as high blood pressure, indigestion, constipation, infertility and others. Whatever is happening in one level of reality (physical, mental, or emotional) also happens in all other levels. Here again, "as above, so below" becomes apparent as external and internal environments are manifested. We experience all of it at all times, at all places.

Even when we think we are making progress with certain aspects in our lives, chances are we have to go back to the core (viscera) and find courage to confront issues affecting our survival. Instead of the habitual response of fight or flight, we transform the disease by creating what we call a dance with the diwata as shared by a hilot. Before you study martial arts or any art form, it is important to initiate a relationship or balance with the fight or flight response which is the diwata of our core. Then we learn to work with the 'butterflies' (fluttery feelings) in our stomach.

As a hilot, through the dance, I help to balance the fight or flight (avoiding) response at the core and connective tissue as a foundation to move forward. With a hilot, the dance is created in sessions. In this dance, you get to know your shortcomings. You have the opportunity to open up the energies necessary for survival, security, grounding and transformation. Through this dance, you can potentially create, re-create and awaken processes of new connections inside and outside your body.

The mystery, better known as 'my story' in this dance is rooted in birth, and the creation of life itself, which is the beginning of transformation. Nature does not make mistakes. We have to understand this process and dance with it. How we can understand this mystery is simply to look and own our personal stories. As my teacher said, "Mystery is nothing but 'my story'. What's my story? My story is my purpose." My role as a hilot is to facilitate your transformation and define your story.

Filipino hilot honors communications and guidance from all diwata through the interplay of four key elements—earth, air, fire and water—found in our bodies and in our environment. We are immersed in these elements as a microcosm. As key elements interact with each other, other elements are formed: metal, crystal, sand, smoke, dust, dew, rock, steam, and clay.

On the next page is an illustration that depicts the play.

The Healing Dance

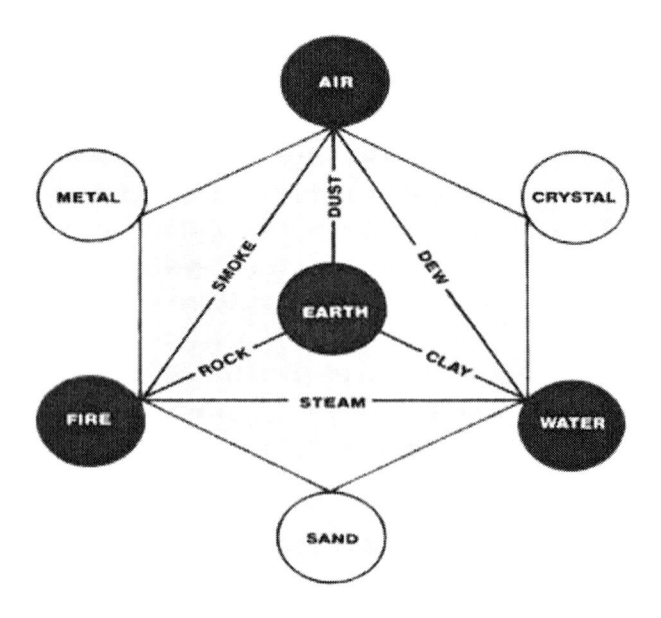

Source: Apostol, V. M. (2010). *Way of the ancient healer: Sacred teachings from the Philippine ancestral traditions.* Berkeley, Calif: North Atlantic Books.

What's important to understand is that these elements influence our beings. You can see their interplay like a chess game. If you make one move, the entire game changes. What do we do when we encounter a change? We are invited to play the game of adaptability, and the game continues. The changes and processes then unfold into behaviours, health conditions and other manifestations that create our stories.

These elements are not isolated from one another, neither are the plants, animals and other beings. The interactions, the play, the dance, and the symphony create infinite possibilities and opportunities for intimacy, for healing and growth. Let us begin with ourselves to know that these key elements are nature's way of governing our becoming or being. When we chose certain food, certain herbs or certain therapy for our disease, we just do not look at it on the physical, chemical or scientific properties but we go deep and beyond.

From below is the earth element which is substance. It manifests as persistence, and endurance. Fire is the element of will and power. It manifests in the energy to achieve. Air is the element of freedom. It manifests in the ability to detach from worldly concerns, thereby finding peace and freedom. The last key element is water, which is change and manifests in adaptability: adapting to anything and everything, and having a deep sense of community that holds all together in any difficulty.

These elements and cycles contribute to ongoing exchanges of energies for balance and harmony with every being. Simply put, these elements, these interactions, these processes are taking place inside and outside of our bodies following transformative cycles of conception, birth, maturity, reflection, and back to conception. Take for example the butterfly that goes from an egg to a larva to a cocoon and to birth. When we understand where we are in the cycle, we have a better understanding of what we need to do next that is in alignment with what's next. It is also worth remembering that these stages in the cycle occur every moment in our lives.

Our stories are the manifestations of the elements like threads that weave patterns that could either be helpful to us or destructive. Just as the diwata are there to help us, within us lies the ultimate creator of our stories.

We can dance through our uncertainties to weave and design our lives. What, how, when, why and where we weave our woven patterns will determine how strong or how long it will last. Will it get through the hard times? This is crucial to keep in mind when looking for solutions to our health conditions or when we want to change our realities, to evolve instead of revolt, and to grow and be humble. This is the dance that reveals the pattern of the tapestry of our lives. This is how nature works. This is how diwata works.

To understand further, I had to ask the question on diwata and its origin from my teacher and healer, African Nganga (shaman) Baba Akinyele Onisegun Karade. This is what he said:

> *Traditionally, diwata (forces in nature) are part of our folklore and cultural experience that's beyond history or mystery "my story". It is "the story." They are the stories made up of characters, forces or electromagnetic energy that our ancestors were very aware of. These forces or superheroes as told to children in nature, represent or make up our very existence. Our ancestors understand the massiveness of Creation and set forth the expression "the creator."*
>
> *This expression represented the whole of its parts called Creation and in this expression we can experience all of creation through the creatures. These creatures, maybe as small as an invisible organism or as big as a very visible hurricane, are all the different expression of the created life on plants. The power or key to our existence is how we define this reality. It's like a fish in the ocean. Do you think that a fish can know the massiveness of the ocean and all that's in it? This is why as children the elders encourage creativity, imagination, adaptability, strength, fortitude, compassion, balance and harmony with a gentle character. A child hearing the stories of these forces or superheroes would become motivated, excited and imaginatively behave like one.*

The Healing Dance

The stories of these superheroes are mostly told by respected elders or initiates in the culture who have earned the rites of passage to infuse the imagination, creativity and wisdom.

Children embrace the stories of superheroes and forces in nature wanting to become the respected elders as well as respecting elders who embody this great power and responsibility. This motivates and prepares them for the rites of passage, a process of intense training to become a respected elder or initiate in the culture.

These superheroes or forces were said to live in, around or about us. Helping to identify our reality, get through hard times and make us aware of how to use our strengths to overcome our weaknesses, building a balance and gentle character, harmony (not dominion) but respect for ourselves first, and then with that which exist in, around and about us. Out of that respect and conditioning comes great power. It is only then that you can truly identify and understand the dualities in nature and how to make balance and call on our strength to overcome our weakness.

Those who become respected elders or initiates have the power to teach, call on or embody wisdom of these forces or superheroes. They live and exist in everything: plant, animal, insect, earth, water, air and fire. All that exist all that Is: visible or invisible.

In some areas of the world like the Philippines, they are called diwata. In other places they may be referred to as angels, deities, gods (guides) or even saints. In the western hemisphere of Africa, the cradle of creation, the identification of these forces or superheroes are extensive. They are identified as Orishas.

Orisha is a combination of two words: Ori (spark of human consciousness) and sha (potentiality of that consciousness). Orisha symbolizes human expression of a particular consciousness and its potentiality. It is a manifestation of divine power in human essence.

You can imagine it as the electromagnetic dance like weaves in fabric that holds it all together. That Divine Presence is what the Kongolese call Simbi: that energy that holds everything together or holds everything up. This dance opens up to infinite possibilities and potentialities. Maintaining Iwa-pele, another West Afrikan practice, means a balance of characters and attitudes – the connection between one's consciousness (Ori) and awareness to one's behaviour.

In Southeast Asia, this dance is identified in the chakras in yoga. Chakras are electromagnetic fields that exist inside the body and coordinates with the electromagnetic field in and around mother earth, 'That holds it together or that holds it up'. This process is influenced by how we respond to our environment, an environment in which children are most vulnerable. This affects childhood habits that determine if the child becomes a respected elder or not.

Children naturally play (dance) and explore their characters and attitudes that exist within them called chakras or Ori-shas, developing their awareness, consciousness, and possibilities. They further develop habits and behaviors contributory to health and wellness, as well as bring order in any given situation most particularly in chaotic situations. This is why letting go and living in the present creates an Iwa-pele balance of characters and attitudes. When always holding on the past (your teacher) or the future (your dream) you'll lose the present (the gift), also known as Simbi, The Divine Presence.

Here's a diagram of chakra and Orishas.

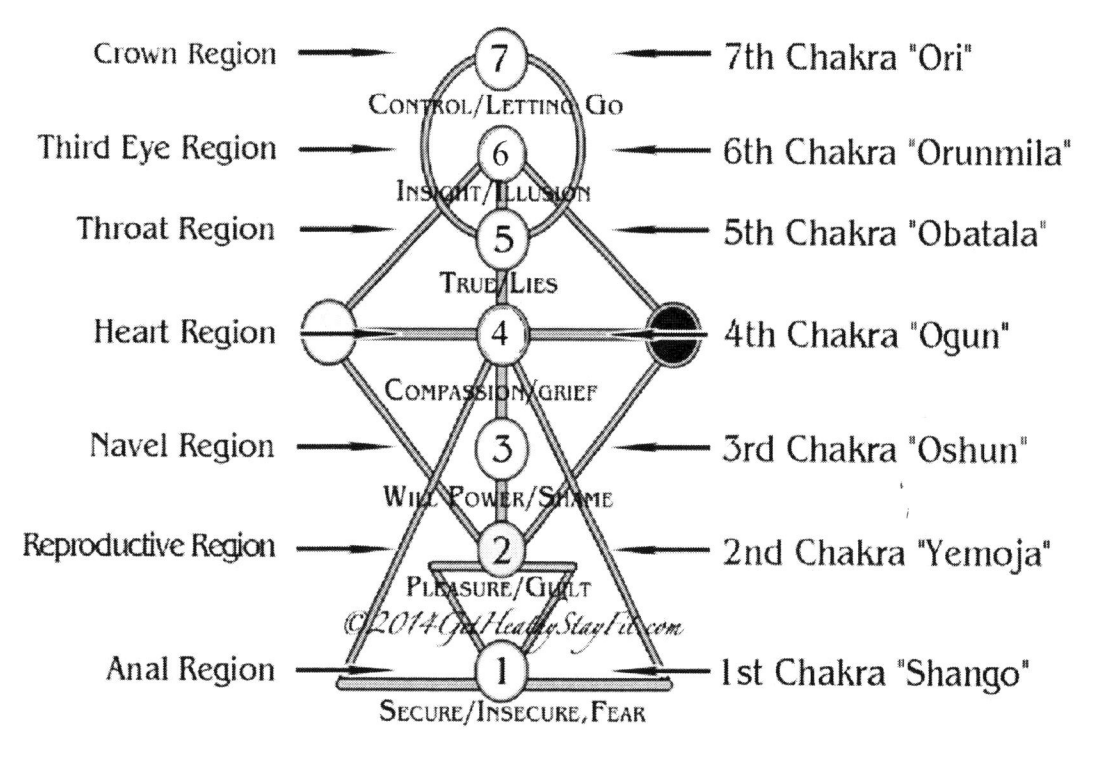

Crown Region	7th Chakra "Ori"	Control/Letting Go
Third Eye Region	6th Chakra "Orunmila"	Insight/Illusion
Throat Region	5th Chakra "Obatala"	True/Lies
Heart Region	4th Chakra "Ogun"	Compassion/Grief
Navel Region	3rd Chakra "Oshun"	Will Power/Shame
Reproductive Region	2nd Chakra "Yemoja"	Pleasure/Guilt
Anal Region	1st Chakra "Shango"	Secure/Insecure, Fear

Source: Akinyele Onisegun Karade, www.gethealthystayfit.com

It is good to remember that you can be the teacher, be the dream, be the present and be the story. My friend, Two Feathers, native of Turtle Island (North America) once said to me, "If you face the sun, you will not see your shadow." The shadow is the ghost that influences disease state. There is nothing to fear but fear itself. The origin of fear isn't dark or void but full to the brim and spills like the cup that runneth over.

The Healing Dance

Recipes   Paraan ng Pagluluto

One summer after visiting the Philippines, an American friend said to me, "Two things I learned about Filipinos: One, they do not mind being close to each other. Two, whenever there is a gathering, there's food."

This is indeed true, not just for Filipinos but all Asian people. We are raised to be generous and caring by sharing food. It does not matter if you have only little to share or if the person next to you is a friend or not. If a visitor arrives at the regular mealtime of the family, there is always plate for the visitor. Friendship and good food go hand in hand. The same is true with space. The size of the house does not stop people from visiting. The host will always offer a space to sleep, even if it means sleeping on the floor for either the guest or the host. To partake in each other's food and space opens up a relationship that expands and strengthens friendship.

I am blessed to have Filipino friends with whom I have shared food and space so that we can bond with each other. The food we shared at work and on other occasions helped us to be healthy and be happy. Sharing in good times enables us to share in bad times.

The recipes contributed by my Filipino friends to this book are similar to those enjoyed by Thai people. Even though we are separated by land and water, traditions are similar. Through indigenous healing foods you may feel at home away from home.

I continue to experience for myself, my family and my clients the power of certain foods as medicine. I offer you cultural food recipes in the context of Filipino-Asian healing arts that eating with mindfulness provides signals to our bodies for optimum health.

Please enjoy the recipes. Have fun in the preparation and savor the taste.

Kumain na po tayo (Let's eat)!

Sweet Coconut Soup   Ginataan

    Traditionally, this tasty, creamy and filling dish is very popular in any social gathering in most Asian countries. This can be enjoyed for breakfast, mirienda (snack) and especially in the afternoon when everyone has just woken up from their siesta, or when others have been working on the rice field. As you hold the bowl of freshly cooked coconut soup, imagine both friends and strangers around you—some sitting while others are squatting on a bamboo porch of a nipa thatched hut. Or you could be sitting on a log with your feet on the dirt road. The chickens are running around the coconut trees. The rice fields are swaying. The summer breeze is blowing on your sweaty face. Is it hot for you? Wait for the dish to cool off. The ginger and anise in it will cool your body at some point in time.

    Ginataan has a special place in my heart. A huge pot of ginataan on top of 3 big rocks with burning flame from firewood was prepared for me on my last days in the Philippines. Community representatives of parents, children and other individuals from the various poor urban and rural places where I worked as a nurse and community organizer gave me a wonderful paalam (goodbye) through ginataan and singing with the accompaniment of guitar. They were wishing me a rich, colorful, wonderful and stable life in United States as they themselves will continue the works of indigenous healing as we all had shared with one another.

    Ginataan has also been ritually prepared for people who have imbalances such as fever, colds, joint problems, inflammations, indigestion, gas/colic pain, heartburn, sore throat, fatigue, hot flashes and many more discomforts both short term and long term. Prepare it with a prayer of thanksgiving and good intention.

    To better invoke the healing powers, stir constantly in one direction only. Stir it clockwise. You want to be in harmony with the vibrations of the spirits of the plant kingdom represented in this dish. As you stir, the steam and aroma will travel to pay homage to the Creator and the spirits. Physically it will prevent the dish from settling at the bottom of the pot and burning.

    All ingredients can be adjusted as desired to suit one's taste and preferences. The adjustment of the quantity of the coconut milk will make a difference in creaminess and consistency. Water can also be added instead of milk, and the amount of cubed ingredients will make it more or less filling. Different amounts of spices will also bring different flavors. Rice syrup, maple syrup or agave can also be used as a natural sweetener. This recipe is wide open for your personal taste preferences.

Ingredients:
5 cups of coconut milk (1 cup should be set aside)
1 cup of pure water
2/3 cup of coconut sugar
1 tablespoon of anise seeds
1 tablespoon of grated ginger root
1 tablespoon of vanilla flavor
1/3 cup of sweet potato or yam in cubes
1/3 cup of cassava in cubes
1/3 cup of yucca in cubes
1 cup of ripe plantain in cubes
1 cup of cooked tapioca balls
Optional: 1/3 cup of fresh, ripe jackfruit in slices
      1 tablespoon of fresh cardamom
      2 tablespoons of grated turmeric

How to prepare:

In a casserole pot, pour 1 cup of pure water, 4 cups of coconut milk, cassava, yucca, and sweet potato or yam. Stir clockwise and let boil. Add the plantain. Stir again and let it boil until everything is soft. Approximately 10 minutes. Add anise, ginger, vanilla, tapioca, and jackfruit. Stir and let boil until everything is tender Approximately 5 minutes. Add coconut sugar. Stir and let boil. Top the dish with the remaining coconut milk. Stir, cover the pot and turn off the flame.

Serve after 7 minutes.

Frequent stirring is advised in order to cook everything evenly and to avoid burning at the bottom.

Makes 5-7 servings for average appetite.

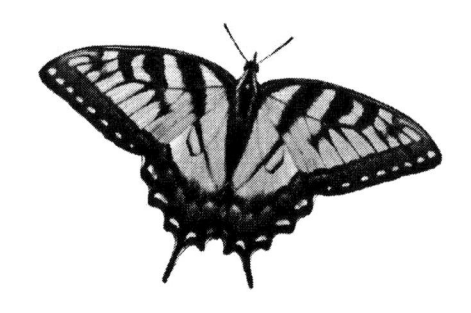

Rice Noodles   Bihon

Noodles represent long and prosperous life. This is why Asian families prepare noodles frequently, particularly during wedding and birthday celebrations. In many Asian countries, particularly Thailand, wide rice noodles are preferred. Filipinos love thin rice noodles. I like them both.

I fondly remember the times that my friends looked forward to going to restaurants with rice noodles as the specialty. It was everyone's favorite dish to share, so it is difficult to say no to an invitation for an afternoon treat of rice noodles. I would save money to be able to eat out and enjoy the company of friends. The rice noodles in one particular restaurant were topped with fresh chopped scallions, mixed with tasty shiitake mushrooms and fresh lemon or lime slices on the side to complete the taste just before we savored it in our mouths. The fresh lemon aroma made the dish even more appetizing. We would order it with warm toasted bread. It may sound as if were eating too many carbohydrates, but none of us gained weight. It is commonly enjoyed at mirienda (snack) time; however, if it is served at mealtime, we enjoy it just the same

This dish can be prepared either as a stir-fry or as a soup. For the first preference, cooking it just before it is served, makes it tastier since the moistness of the dish remains unchanged. Once it cools off, it tends to be dry, but even when it is cold, the taste remains because of the blending of spices. The softness of the noodles gives your mouth a soothing texture as you slurp the soup. This is especially true when you are ill with colds, fever, upset stomach, fatigue, weaknesses and other ailments.

Ingredients:
5 small packs of thin rice noodles (sold at Oriental or health food stores.)
1 cup thinly sliced shiitake mushrooms
1 cup thinly sliced carrots
1 cup sliced cabbage
1 cup snow peas
1 I cup thinly sliced celery
1 cup thinly sliced onions
2 cups tofu in cubes (marinated in natural soy sauce or liquid amino and balsamic vinegar for fifteen minutes If desired, chicken, beef, pork or shrimp can be used instead or in addition.)
5 crushed garlic cloves
5 tablespoons cold-pressed coconut oil for stir-frying
5 tablespoons natural soy sauce or liquid amino (available at the health food stores)

1 cup chopped cilantro (Chinese parsley)
1 cup chopped scallions (for topping) Three slices of lemon (for serving on the side)
3 cups of distilled or spring water

How to prepare:

Place 3 tablespoons of safflower oil in a wok. Add tofu cubes and stir fry lightly until browned. Add onions, garlic and ginger and cook for a minute or two till lightly brown. Add the shiitake, carrots, celery, and cabbage and stir-fry for three minutes. Add the snow peas and cilantro (Chinese parsley) and stir-fry for three minutes. Set aside 1/3 of the above stir-fried vegetables. Add 3 cups of distilled or spring water, soy sauce or liquid amino to the remaining 2/3, stir, cover and boil. Add the noodles, stir and cook until the noodles are tender. Approximately five minutes. Serve on a big dish. Top with scallions and the remaining stir-fried vegetables.

Place the slices of lemons on the side of the platter. If everyone likes lemon on their noodles, the host can squeeze the lemon and sprinkle the juice on the noodles after everyone have taken their seats or leave the lemons for the guests to squeeze on their individuals plates. Place extra soy sauce on the table.

Makes 7 average amount of servings.

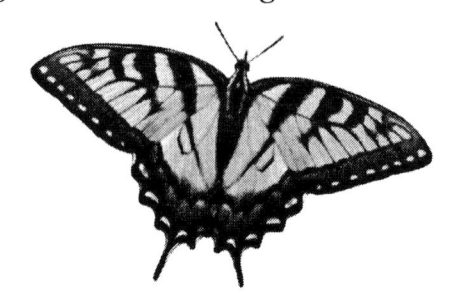

Vegetable Spring Roll
Lumpiang Gulay

I have not met anyone who does not like lumpia (spring roll). It is a very common dish at home and for social gatherings. To the person who decides to make this dish, I know that one must have a tremendous love for cooking and an abundance of patience, kindness and generosity in one's heart.

One must make time from the beginning until the setting of the dish. Artistic ability must be called upon in wrapping the vegetables. Once they are wrapped, deep fried and set on the table or individual dishes, it becomes a beautiful gift-wrapped food that sates your palate to bring you closer to the cook/artist who might be a friend or a prospective friend.

I am so touched when someone makes spring rolls especially for me. The energy that one needs to prepare this dish makes it a gift beyond appetite. It is caring and friendship molded into the art and love of cooking and sharing.

My mother used to make hundreds of lumpia every day and supply the canteens/cafeterias of various high schools, colleges and universities in our area. It was a tedious job that I didn't feel like doing my best at. I had a lot of rejects, so my mother did not ask me to help her often. My younger sister was so patient and was extremely good at wrapping rolls so neatly and artistically that she helped my mother more than I. Am I a trickster or what?

With our fingers we savor this dish for mirienda (snack), as an appetizer or as part of the meal. When served hot, it is very delicious. This is highly recommended in any illness that decreases one's appetite especially during febrile conditions. Always prepare it with the spirit of thanksgiving. Be one with the Creator.

Ingredients:
For the roll:
1 cup thinly sliced bamboo shoots (available at Oriental store)
1 cup thinly sliced shiitake mushrooms
1 cup thinly sliced carrots
1 cup thinly sliced cabbage
1 cup thinly sliced celery
1 cup thinly sliced onions
1 cup mung bean sprouts
1 cup cooked mung bean noodles
1 cup thinly sliced sweet potato
1 cup tofu in cubes (marinated for fifteen minutes in natural soy sauce or liquid amino and balsamic vinegar. If preferred, chicken, beef, pork or shrimps can be used instead or in addition.)
5 cloves of garlic, crushed

3 tablespoons shredded ginger root
Cold pressed coconut oil for stir frying and deep frying
3 tablespoons natural soy sauce or liquid amino (available at Health Food stores)
12-15 spring roll wrappers (available at Oriental stores)

For the sauce:
1 cup coconut vinegar (or apple cider vinegar)
7 garlic cloves, crushed
1.5 tablespoons agave or 3 tablespoons of coconut sugar or 2 tablespoons maple syrup or 2 tablespoons honey

How to prepare:
    Mix all the ingredients for the sauce, shake it in a bottle and set aside. Shake it every now and then as you continue to prepare the roll. Shake it just before you pour it into individual small shallow bowls or place it in a jar where friends can use it as they please, once the lumpia is deep fried and ready to be put on the table.
    In a wok, stir-fry the marinated tofu until lightly brown. Set aside on a platter to cool off. In the same wok, stir-fry the onions, garlic and ginger until lightly brown. Add sweet potatoes and carrots. Stir and cover for a minute. Add cabbage, bamboo shoots and mushrooms, then stir and cover for one minute. Add celery, stir, and cover for one minute. Add the rest of the ingredients except for the tofu that was set aside, stir, cover and cool off.
    Once everything is cool, follow the instructions on how to use the wrappers, according to the package. Add the desired number of pieces of tofu per roll. Neatly fold the corners of each wrapper so no vegetables will fall out. It is easier to manage when preparing small to medium-sized rolls.
    Deep-fry on hot oil until brown. Once a roll is fried, let it stand on an angle to drip dry onto a paper towel or dish. Do not put rolls on top of each other. They will get squashed, especially when they start to cool. Serve hot.
    Makes 12-15 medium size lumpia

Poems

Tula

In this section there are poems that I have written as well as two that were written as gifts for me. I hope that you enjoy them.

POETRY IN MOTION

This is the moment that you and I create.
To touch, flow, breathe as we generate.
Whispers of wind, I enter and leave you,
To graciously ascend and descend
This bayou seed develops
Stores, transforms, grows and absorbs.
Giving you my body, heart and soul,
That I may feel and listen to the depth of yours.
It isn't just me that makes a difference.
You and I
Create a harmony in divergence.
Journey of vibrations in
Human rivers of love potion,
Resonating
Unity
Of verses in motion.

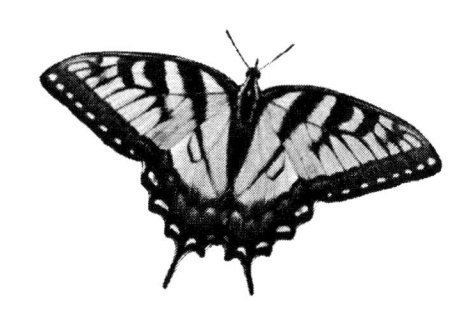

LOVE THYSELF

Too many times we
End up complaining, "I do not experience enough loving."
Work seems endless
Problems countless
Time passes us by
We know not why
For once in thy life, take a break in thy strife
Indulge in indigenous massage
And breakdown the facade
From thy weary feet,
To thine heart so beat
Ancient blend of presses,
Rhythmic motions as spices
Guide the mindful giver
Protect the receiver.
Experience the power
Divine energy as thy lover
Exotic goddess
From heavens high
Amazing souls
In web intertwine
Everything joins in one
Inside and outside.
Meditative healing art
Right on our side.
Mindfulness is healing
Sen energies opening.
Compassion and loving
Thine heart overflowing

A TRIBUTE TO MY ANIMAL GUIDES

On the east, I thank the frog for singing
That I may call upon the rains, and all the waters
So I can purify my health and continue vibrating.
On the south, I thank the antelope for actions
That taught me to move with pace and grace
And never to waste, but survive in motions.
On the west, I thank the lizard for dreaming
That allowed me to travel across the moon and stars,
With my fears and hopes as I stop resisting.
On the north, I thank the alligator for integration
That I accept each moment as an opportunity
With no judgments, nor worries, but only assimilation.
From above, I thank the salmon for wisdom and inner knowing
That I respect my perceptions and remain grounded in currents
For within me are hidden resources of learning.
From below, I thank the blue heron for self-reflection
That I discover my gifts, emotions and thoughts
I am woven in the Great Spirit's connection.
From within, I thank the hummingbird for joy
That my presence brings people together in sweet relationships
So they can thrive in beauty and succulent nectar of life.
On my right side, I thank the cricket for communication
That I listen with my soul so vibrations resonate
And with earth's music we divinely connect.
On my left side, I thank the deer for gentleness
That I may touch the hearts and minds of wounded beings
And bring us compassion and loving kindness.

IN MY HANDS

I am the nurse who makes the difference,
I am the nurse who sets the preference,
I am the nurse who makes the sacrifice,
I am the nurse who gives wise advice.
I am...because, YOU and I...In my hands!
With patience of a tiny ant, I take part in organizing,
Full of wolf's creative ideas and keen understanding.
Contented without preconceptions or suspicions,
Sensitive to all accomplishments and perceptions.
Innovative leadership grows in my hands!

Like an eagle I will soar high for more,
In the huge magnet earth, I am the core,
Solidly grounded and rooted to my being.
I take the flame that molds my becoming,
Caterpillar transforms right in my hands!

In darkness, I see through your faces,
In silence, I listen to your phrases,
Astounded, myself is in the middle,
Of egotistic minds that are fickle.
Loving kindness streams in my hands!

In the cycle of adversities
I give all to responsibilities,
Praise and honor for a job well done.
Inner strength is never gone.
Rainbow of Peace shines in my hands!

Gentleness is always there for me to share —
My turtle shell will keep me safe if you dare,
Wings of my soul on purpose with the Divine,
In the realm of spirit I am fine.
Creator's healing is in my hands!

> *Lovingly dedicated to all the nurses who have gone before me who continue to carry the torch, and the future ones who are willing to inherit the legacy.*

MY GOODNESS GRACIOUS

An iron fist named Grace...
Trance dancing in a velvet glove,
Hiding quietly shining precious stones,
Set in solar gold and silver finger rings that sparkle rainbow.
Like her joyous goddess smile...
She swims at midnight full moons,
Naked like the dark soft skin,
Of the night sky laughing.
Through her son's love for his mother's free-spirited journey...
Her big graceful heart embraces,
The world as her soul mate...
The black earth with gentle love energy.
Of her Filipino ancestors dancing...
Where spirits ride the breath wind,
Of her Madonna image breast feeding,
Her white haired wisdom child...
Through the dark tipped nipples
Of her Milky Way powers...
She sings unspoken dance melodies
With her magic sounds that manifest
As in her unconditional love heart.
"So be it"
Hang it there my sister....
I got your back.
Onepeaceluv,

Your brother Jamal
January 24, 2001

HER HANDS...

It is not just a massage that day.
It is more the benefit and the way.
She teaches various hands in many lands.
And passionately imparts in everyone's heart.
It is not just how her hands feel.
It is much more how her hands heal.
It is not just pleasure you will find.
It is much more the peace of mind.

Herb, 1998

What's Next?   Ano ang Susunod?

I hope I have inspired you to look at your journey in a way that's empowering to you, knowing that health and well-being is simple, doable, accessible and sustainable. There are cultural ways of healing that you can draw from like a money market account that has a constant positive balance with interest earnings that gets reinvested in your health account. After all, your best investment is your optimum health and well-being.

Speaking as an immigrant nurse, the influx of migrant workers from various traditions is causing significant cultural exchange and influence around the world. As direct consumers of fast-changing technology, we have non-stop interactions, whether we choose it or not, to be close to one another in one way, and yet distant in another. Internet and mobile exchanges of communications have become the standard business and family affairs. We have our social media friends. We feel we belong to something greater than ourselves. Yet, we are faced with health conditions even at an early age, such as depression, crimes of hatred and violence, we have not seen before. Many feel disconnected from social and emotional support. Many live in compartmentalized and fragmented lives that make it difficult to see the wholeness and sense of greater purpose of our existence. What do we do? Where do we go from here? What does tomorrow bring for each of us?

Indigenous healing is a ritual that embodies everything that made it to be what it was before and what it is now. This brings intense satisfaction, love and compassion. Oftentimes, we look for ways to better our society and ourselves, when all we have to do is to live on the sacredness of teachings and rituals in indigenous healing. Rituals have connected many generations to the sun, the moon, the stars, the plants, the animals, the water and the land as we sleep and wake up, by day and by night, as we ascend and descend, in dry and wet seasons.

Everything is medicine. Life is like an ocean with ripples that manifest inside and outside our bodies. I would like to continue the dance by being a partner with those who are ready to transform their authentic healing journeys. Together, this dance will form a tapestry of woven patterns of healing ways responsive to the needs of individuals, families, communities and nations. We will explore cultural ways of knowing what works and find health sustainability whenever and wherever we can. We will encourage dialogues to continue as we share our stories so that others may be inspired to live in harmony with diwata.

It is my joy to share the profound tapestry of indigenous healing. When we remain open to the experience, wonders happen. These arts are more than a pattern of techniques, more than a dance, more than a poem and more than a weave. They create a dynamic story of being and the becoming of people, culture and philosophy. They may have been cultivated in the past, but they are as responsive in the present as they were in the past. Through these arts, the value of external forces to evoke internal change is revealed.

I look forward to the future when I can tell you more stories on how indigenous healing arts are applied to current situations for those who choose that route. Although ancient, Filipino hilot is still relevant today. I will continue to find more voice for diwata in writing, in conversations, and in movements for transformation.

Ang kapayapaan ay sumainyo! (Peace be with you!)

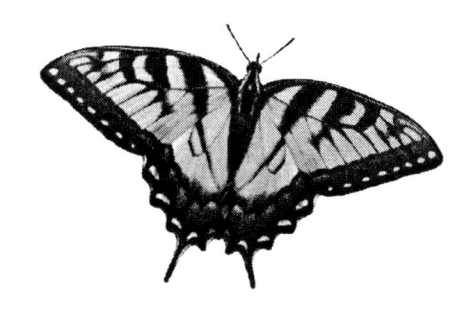

References

Mga sanggunian

Apostol, V. M. (2010). Way of the Ancient Healer: Sacred teachings from the Philippine ancestral traditions. Berkeley, Calif: North Atlantic Books.

Baet, A. S. (2001). Harimaw Buno : the art of Filipino wrestling. Philippines?: s.n.].

Capoeira, N. (2002). Capoeira : roots of the dance-fight-game. Berkeley, Calif.: North Atlantic Books.

Gach, M. R. (1990). Acupressure's potent points : a guide to self-care for common ailments. New York: Bantam Books.

Judith, A. (1999). Wheels of life : a user's guide to the chakra system. St. Paul, Minn.: Llewellyn Publications.

Kaptchuk, T. J. (1983). The web that has no weaver : understanding Chinese medicine. New York: Congdon & Weed : distributed by St. Martin's Press.

Kunz, K. K. B. S. K. L. (1982). The complete guide to foot reflexology. Englewood Cliffs, N.J.: Prentice-Hall.

Lad, V. (1984). Ayurveda : the science of self-healing : a practical guide. Santa Fe, N.M.: Lotus Press.

Lambert, A. S. C. I. o. T. M. U. S. A. (1994). The traditional massage of Thailand Thai I basic workshop : teaching the front position with Arthur Lambert. Boynton Beach, FL: IMS-USA.

Lundberg, P. (2003). The book of shiatsu : a complete guide to using hand pressure and gentle manipulation to improve your health, vitality, and stamina. New York: Simon & Schuster.

Mehta, S. M. M. M. S. (1990). Yoga : the Iyengar way. New York: A.A. Knopf.

Pastor-Roces, M. B. D. T. W. (1991). Sinaunang habi : Philippine ancestral weave. [Quezon City, Philippines]: N. Coseteng.

Sams, J., Carson, D., & Werneke, A. C. (1999). Medicine cards. New York: St. Martin's Press.

Shapiro, M. M. (1997). The Dancing Meditation of Thailand Traditional Massage. Newton, MA: Acupuncture & Healing Therapies.

Sieg, K. W. A. S. P. S. A. D. C. D. (1985). Illustrated essentials of musculoskeletal anatomy. Gainesville, Fla.: Megabooks.

Sulite, E. G. (1986). The Secrets of Arnis. San Juan, Philippines: Socorro Publications.

Vanzant, I. (1996). Faith in the valley: lessons for women on the journey toward peace. New York: Simon & Schuster.

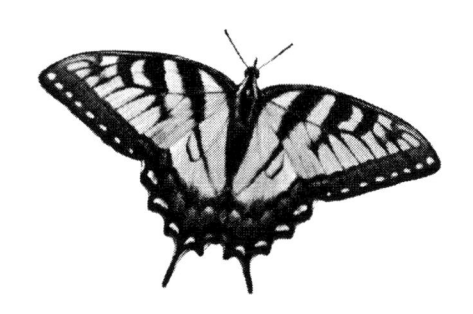

About Grace

Tungkol kay Grace

Grace Sunga Asagra MA, RN, HN-BC, HC-BC, is a traditional Filipino hilot (indigenous health practitioner using joint-muscular manipulations, bentusa, cooking and herbal foods), holistic health coach (nutritionist-counselor-life coach-health advocate), author and speaker on "Who and What's the Matter with You." A seasoned nurse with over 20 years of critical care nursing, she was a barefoot nurse in Legaspi City, Philippines, organizing and empowering locals to use natural resources for sustainable health solutions.

Currently, her practice as a hilot is the dance co-created with mga diwata (forces in nature/deities/angels) and mga ninuno (ancestors). She guides individuals to change the course of their health from chronic conditions to healthy aging through understanding the dance between their inner and outer selves.

Grace specializes in optimum health and wellness programs in partnership with clients who want to weave authentic, integrative, functional, ancestral and traditional health solutions into improving overall holistic health. Some of the success stories that inspire her include a nine-year-old girl in the Philippines with history of cerebral palsy who was able walk again after series of hilot sessions, a sixty-year-old female business owner who lost thirty pounds with improved clinical changes and was able to discontinue her blood pressure medication, with her doctor's approval. Also a seventy-six-year-old male college professor who experienced healthier prostate conditions without prescription medications and a fifty-six-year old female with history of colon cancer who chose not to have surgery and became cancer free to much surprise of her oncologist.

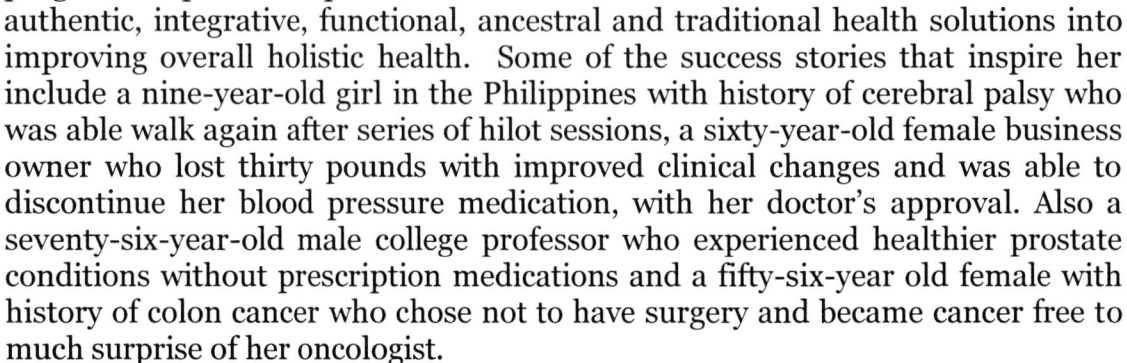

Grace's caring ways and healing embody respect for a person's bio-individuality, authenticity and wholeness through healthcare programs that support an environment for optimum healthy gene expression founded on her relationship with her clients and diwata, bringing about awareness and responsibility to her clients' health and well-being, as well as holism embodied in cultural ways of knowing and being to express inherent healing ways. She honors all experiences and trusts the process as medicine and healing in collaboration with those who join her in this journey. Learn more about her at her websites, www.graceasagra.com and www.filipinohilot.com.

About the Shaman

Akinyele Onisegun Karade was born David Stanley to parents whose lineage runs beyond slavery in South Carolina to chief healers in West Afrika. His great grandparents' legacy guided and protected him as he walked his path in response to the call of his healing power and practice. His ancestors had provided him the training and experiences to help him, other individuals and groups through difficult situations in physical, mental, emotional or spiritual wellness.

Akinyele apprenticed with Dr. George Zofchak, herbalist, chiropractor and Naturopath of Tatra Herb Company, one of the pioneers in the herbal industry, established in 1929 in Morrisville, Pennsylvania. He is an advanced shiatsu practitioner and studied at The International School of Shiatsu with an orientation in acupuncture and traditional Oriental Medicine and is a Certified Hydrotherapist. He has also studied "Hobo medicine" at the famous Tree of Life Center in Harlem and has been initiated as a priest in the Yoruba culture.

As a traditional health practitioner for over 30 years, Akinyele has worked with physicians, dentists, teachers, chiropractors, yoga teachers, massage professionals, professional athletes and a wide variety of people of all ages, genders and ancestral traditions. His way of integrating shiatsu and SijuAse, his own original techniques, help people to relax, quiet their minds, help improve their breathing, improve range of motion, relieve pains and recover from serious ailments. He is the founder of SijuAse (opening, moving and adaptability and self-awareness of life force). More information on him may be found at www.GetHealthyStayFit.com.

About the Photographer

Ricardo Barros has worked as a photographer, curator and teacher for over thirty years. His works are in the permanent collections of ten museums, including: The Smithsonian Museum of American Art, The Fogg Art Museum, Museu de Arte de São Paulo (MASP), Museu da Imagem e do Som (MIS), and the Philadelphia Museum of Art. His award-winning book, "Facing Sculpture: A Portfolio of Portraits, Sculpture, and Related Ideas," has been hailed by critics as "a work beyond categories." Barros received a Fellowship in Photography from the New Jersey State Council on the Arts in 1984 His website is www.ricardobarros.com.

About the Cover

The Painting: Babaylan by Artist: Art Zamora

BABAYLAN, the cover of this manuscript, is courtesy of Art Zamora, a well-known Filipino artist whose many art works are in the hands of public and private collectors around the world. The original Babaylan painting is currently on display at the author's residence in Princeton, New Jersey.

Babaylan is a Filipino word for a mystical healer found in different tribes in the Philippine Islands. The healer's culture, traditions, beliefs, grace and power are used to treat various illnesses. Prayers, chanting, herbs, dances and sacred rituals are associated with this healing. Time seems to stop and for a moment we get a glimpse into the future and the mysteries of the universe. Is it infinity? Is it eternity? Is it just another moment?

Art Zamora uses a highly personal approach by employing the image of the babaylan with an almost metaphysical feeling. Its color and form achieve a splendid balance between subject matter and composition.

His passion is painting. He developed, explored and innovated his artistic talents in oils, acrylics and watercolor paintings. His Oriental background and his Western experience as a world-class jewelry designer influenced his strokes. Nature, with its colors of mysticism and glory, is depicted frequently in his works. He can best be described as a cross between a modified realist and an impressionist.

He has had numerous solo art and group exhibitions around the world. He was the founder of the Concerned Artists in New Visual Art Style Systems (CANVASS), Art Channel Kapwa-Pilipino (ACKP), and the Association of Filipino Jewelry Designers (AFJED).

His healing experiences with Filipino tribal healers have protected him in his travels. He has always called upon the spirit of the babaylan to enhance his paintings with respect to nature and its healing powers.